T0263560

Advances in Wound and Bone Healing

Guest Editor

ADAM LANDSMAN, DPM, PhD, FACFAS

CLINICS IN PODIATRIC MEDICINE AND SURGERY

www.podiatric.theclinics.com

Consulting Editor
THOMAS ZGONIS, DPM, FACFAS

October 2009 • Volume 26 • Number 4

SAUNDERS an imprint of ELSEVIER, Inc.

W.B. SAUNDERS COMPANY
A Division of Elsevier Inc.

1600 John F. Kennedy Boulevard ● Suite 1800 ● Philadelphia, Pennsylvania 19103-2899

http://www.theclinics.com

CLINICS IN PODIATRIC MEDICINE AND SURGERY Volume 26, Number 4
October 2009 ISSN 0891-8422, ISBN-13: 978-1-4377-1267-4, ISBN-10: 1-4377-1267-3

Editor: Patrick Manley

© 2009 Elsevier ■ All rights reserved.

This journal and the individual contributions contained in it are protected under copyright by Elsevier, and the following terms and conditions apply to their use:

Photocopying

Single photocopies of single articles may be made for personal use as allowed by national copyright laws. Permission of the Publisher and payment of a fee is required for all other photocopying, including multiple or systematic copying, copying for advertising or promotional purposes, resale, and all forms of document delivery. Special rates are available for educational institutions that wish to make photocopies for non-profit educational classroom use. For information on how to seek permission visit www.elsevier.com/permissions or call: (+44) 1865 843830 (UK)/(+1) 215 239 3804 (USA).

Derivative Works

Subscribers may reproduce tables of contents or prepare lists of articles including abstracts for internal circulation within their institutions. Permission of the Publisher is required for resale or distribution outside the institution. Permission of the Publisher is required for all other derivative works, including compilations and translations (please consult www.elsevier.com/permissions).

Electronic Storage or Usage

Permission of the Publisher is required to store or use electronically any material contained in this journal, including any article or part of an article (please consult www.elsevier.com/permissions). Except as outlined above, no part of this publication may be reproduced, stored in a retrieval system or transmitted in any form or by any means, electronic, mechanical, photocopying, recording or otherwise, without prior written permission of the Publisher.

Notice

No responsibility is assumed by the Publisher for any injury and/or damage to persons or property as a matter of products liability, negligence or otherwise, or from any use or operation of any methods, products, instructions or ideas contained in the material herein. Because of rapid advances in the medical sciences, in particular, independent verification of diagnoses and drug dosages should be made.

Although all advertising material is expected to conform to ethical (medical) standards, inclusion in this publication does not constitute a guarantee or endorsement of the quality or value of such product or of the claims made of it by its manufacturer.

Clinics in Podiatric Medicine and Surgery (ISSN 0891-8422) is published quarterly by Elsevier Inc., 360 Park Avenue South, New York, NY 10010-1710. Months of publication are January, April, July, and October. Subscription prices are $229.00 per year for US individuals, $360.00 per year for US institutions, $118.00 per year for US students and residents, $275.00 per year for Canadian individuals, $445.00 for Canadian institutions, $326.00 for international individuals, $445.00 per year for international institutions and $167.00 per year for Canadian and foreign students/residents. To receive student/resident rate, orders must be accompanied by name of affiliated institution, date of term, and the *signature* of program/residency coordinator on institution letterhead. Orders will be billed at individual rate until proof of status is received. Foreign air speed delivery is included in all *Clinics* subscription prices. All prices are subject to change without notice. POSTMASTER: Send address changes to *Clinics in Podiatric Medicine and Surgery*, Elsevier Health Sciences Division, Subscription Customer Service, 3251 Riverport Lane, Maryland Heights, MO 63043. **Customer Service: 1-800-654-2452 (U.S. and Canada); 314-447-8871 (outside U.S. and Canada). Fax: 314-447-8029. E-mail: journalscustomerservice-usa@elsevier.com (for print support); journalsonlinesupport-usa@elsevier.com (for online support).**

Reprints. For copies of 100 or more of articles in this publication, please contact the Commercial Reprints Department, Elsevier Inc., 360 Park Avenue South, New York, NY 10010-1710. Tel.: 212-633-3812; Fax: 212-462-1935; E-mail: reprints@elsevier.com.

Clinics in Podiatric Medicine and Surgery is covered in *MEDLINE/PubMed (Index Medicus)* and *EMBASE/Excerpta Medica.*

Printed and bound by CPI Group (UK) Ltd, Croydon, CR0 4YY

Transferred to Digital Print 2011

CLINICS IN PODIATRIC MEDICINE AND SURGERY

CONSULTING EDITOR
THOMAS ZGONIS, DPM, FACFAS

EDITORIAL BOARD MEMBERS – USA

Babak Baravarian, DPM, FACFAS
Neal M Blitz, DPM, FACFAS
Peter A Blume, DPM, FACFAS
Patrick R Burns, DPM, FACFAS
Alan R Catanzariti, DPM, FACFAS
Luke D Cicchinelli, DPM, FACFAS
Lawrence A DiDomenico, DPM, FACFAS
Lawrence Ford, DPM, FACFAS
Robert G Frykberg, DPM
Jordan P Grossman, DPM, FACFAS
Graham A Hamilton, DPM, FACFAS
Allen M Jacobs, DPM, FACFAS
Gary Peter Jolly, DPM, FACFAS
Molly S Judge, DPM, FACFAS
Adam S Landsman, DPM, PhD, FACFAS
Vincent J Mandracchia, DPM, MHA, FACFAS
Luis E Marin, DPM, FACFAS
Robert W Mendicino, DPM, FACFAS
Samuel S Mendicino, DPM, FACFAS
Thomas S Roukis, DPM, PhD, FACFAS
Laurence G Rubin, DPM, FACFAS
John M Schuberth, DPM
John J Stapleton, DPM, AACFAS
Trent K Statler, DPM, FACFAS
Jerome K Steck, DPM, FACFAS
John S Steinberg, DPM, FACFAS
George F Wallace, DPM, FACFAS
Bruce Werber, DPM, FACFAS
Glenn M Weinraub, DPM, FACFAS
Charles M Zelen, DPM, FACFAS

EDITORIAL BOARD MEMBERS – INTERNATIONAL

Thanos Badekas, MD (Athens, Greece)
Tanil Esemenli, MD (Istanbul, Turkey)
Armin Koller, MD (Muenster, Germany)
Ali Oznur, MD (Ankara, Turkey)
Enrico Parino, MD (Torino, Italy)
Pier Carlo Pisani, MD (Torino, Italy)
Vasilios D Polyzois, MD, PhD, FHCOS (Athens, Greece)
Emmanouil D Stamatis, MD, FHCOS, FACS (Athens, Greece)
Victor Valderrabano, MD, PhD (Basel, Switzerland)

Contributors

CONSULTING EDITOR

THOMAS ZGONIS, DPM, FACFAS
Associate Professor and Chief, Division of Podiatric Medicine and Surgery, Department of Orthopaedic Surgery, Director, Reconstructive Foot and Ankle Fellowship, University of Texas Health Science Center at San Antonio, San Antonio, Texas

GUEST EDITOR

ADAM LANDSMAN, DPM, PhD, FACFAS
Attending Physician and Co-Director of Fellowship Training, Division of Podiatric Surgery, Beth Israel Deaconess Medical Center; Assistant Professor of Surgery, Harvard Medical School Boston, Massachusetts

AUTHORS

RONALD BELCZYK, DPM
Assistant Professor, Department of Orthopaedic Surgery, Division of Podiatric Medicine and Surgery, The University of Texas Health Science Center at San Antonio, San Antonio, Texas

STEPHEN A. BRIGIDO, DPM
Foot and Ankle Center at Coordinated Health, Bethlehem, Pennsylvania

CLAIRE M. CAPOBIANCO, DPM
Fellow, Reconstructive Foot and Ankle Surgery and Clinical Instructor, Department of Orthopaedic Surgery, Division of Podiatric Medicine and Surgery, University of Texas Health Science Center at San Antonio, San Antonio, Texas

EMILY A. COOK, DPM, MPH
Instructor in Surgery, Department of Surgery, Division of Podiatric Surgery, Harvard Medical School, Beth Israel Deaconess Medical Center, Boston, Massachusetts

JEREMY J. COOK, DPM, MPH
Instructor in Surgery, Department of Surgery, Division of Podiatric Surgery, Harvard Medical School, Beth Israel Deaconess Medical Center, Boston, Massachusetts

KEVIN G. CORNWELL, PhD
TEI Biosciences Inc., Boston, Massachusetts

KENNETH S. JAMES, PhD
TEI Biosciences Inc., Boston, Massachusetts

ADAM LANDSMAN, DPM, PhD, FACFAS
Attending Physician and Co-Director of Fellowship Training, Division of Podiatric Surgery, Beth Israel Deaconess Medical Center; Assistant Professor of Surgery, Harvard Medical School Boston, Massachusetts

DAVID L. NIELSON, DPM
Foot and Ankle Associates of Southwest Virginia; Professional Education and Research Institute, Roanoke, Virginia

CRYSTAL L. RAMANUJAM, DPM
Fellow, Postgraduate Research and Clinical Instructor, Department of Orthopaedic Surgery, Division of Podiatric Medicine and Surgery, The University of Texas Health Science Center at San Antonio, San Antonio, Texas

KEVIN RIEMER, DPM
Fellow in Reconstructive Foot Surgery and Research, Harvard Medical School, Division of Podiatric Surgery, Beth Israel Deaconess Medical Center, Boston, Massachusetts

THOMAS M. ROCCHIO, DPM
PA Podiatry; PA Foot and Ankle Associates, Allentown, Pennsylvania; Easton Hospital Wound Healing Center, Easton, Pennsylvania

THOMAS S. ROUKIS, DPM, PhD, FACFAS
Chief of Limb Preservation Service and Director of Limb Preservation Complex; Lower Extremity Surgery and Research Fellowship, Department of Surgery, Vascular/Endovascular Surgery Service, Madigan Army Medical Center, MCHJ-SV, Tacoma, Washington

HAROLD SCHOENHAUS, DPM
Penn-Presbyterian Medical Center, Philadelphia, Pennsylvania

SIMON E. SMITH, BPod, MPod, FACPS
Fellow, Department of Podiatry, Australasian College of Podiatric Surgeons and Musculoskeletal Research Center, La Trobe University, Bundoora, VIC, Australia

BRIAN S. STOVER, DPM
Clinical Research Fellow, Professional Education and Research Institute/SALSA, Roanoke, Virginia

DREW TAFT, DPM
Chief Resident, Harvard Medical School, Division of Podiatric Surgery, Beth Israel Deaconess Medical Center, Boston, Massachusetts

MICHAEL TROIANO, DPM
Penn-Presbyterian Medical Center, Philadelphia, Pennsylvania

CHARLES M. ZELEN, DPM, FACFAS
Podiatry Section Chief, Department of Surgery, Carilion Clinic; Podiatry Section Chief, Department of Orthopaedics, HCA Lewis Gale Hospital; Director of Professional Education and Research Institute; Foot and Ankle Associates of Southwest Virginia, Roanoke, Virginia

THOMAS ZGONIS, DPM, FACFAS
Associate Professor and Chief, Division of Podiatric Medicine and Surgery, Department of Orthopaedics, Director, Reconstructive Foot and Ankle Fellowship, University of Texas Health Science Center at San Antonio, San Antonio, Texas

Contents

> The biological and physical augmentation provided by extracellular matrix (ECM) derived implants continues to challenge and refine the conventional wisdom of biomaterials. It is now appreciated that different tissue-processing methodologies can produce ECM devices with characteristic post-implantation responses ranging from the classic foreign body encapsulation of a permanent implant, to one where the implant is degraded and resorbed, to one where the processed ECM implant is populated by local fibroblasts and supporting vasculature to generate a new, metabolically active tissue (gTissue). This article reviews the multiple ECM devices available clinically and highlights the impact of tissue source and processing on physicomechanical properties and host-implant interactions, with regard to surgical applications and clinical considerations.

> Collagen is one of the fundamental building blocks of skin and plays a critical role in wound healing. This article looks at the wide array of collagen and living skin equivalent products containing collagen and living cells, and at how these may be used in the treatment of diabetic foot ulcers. Solid collagen, foamed collagen, living skin equivalents, and living cadaveric skin are considered. Clinical examples are included, along with a brief discussion of wound dressings that may help to enhance the incorporation of these materials.

> Biologic scaffolds have become an integral part of surgical soft tissue reconstruction in recent years. The increased use of these materials can be partially attributed to poor long-term outcomes with synthetic products as well as the cost and morbidity associated with allografts and autografts. Bioscaffolds can augment natural healing processes of tendons and ligaments while providing additional structural support. Although these

implants lack the mechanical strength of synthetics and other transplants, proper preparation can optimize their load-sharing capacity. This article presents methods that can improve these characteristics of bioscaffolds. Available studies in foot and ankle applications have shown minimal complications in a variety of techniques.

Treatment of plantar fat pad migration and atrophy has caused concern for decades. Patients can present with pain, callus formation, or ulceration. The purpose of this article is to review the results of a consecutive series of patients treated for fat pad atrophy of the plantar foot, using a minimally invasive implantation of an acellular human dermal allograft as a tissue augmentation. This material was chosen for the fat pad supplementation because of previous reports of success in tendon and ligament augmentation, wound healing, and interpositional arthroplasty.

Over the past two decades, autologous platelets that have been sequestered, concentrated, and mixed with thrombin to generate growth factor–concentrated platelet-rich plasma for application to bone and wounds to aide healing have been a subject of great interest. This article reviews the literature related to the use of autologous platelet-rich plasma in bone and wound healing, and reviews the processes necessary to secure a high concentration of viable platelets. Although not yet definitive, autologous platelet-rich plasma has been shown to be safe, reproducible, and effective in mimicking the natural process of bone and wound healing.

In reconstructive foot and ankle surgery, the use of bone graft is common. Whether for trauma, acquired or congenital deformities, arthrodeses, joint replacement, bone loss from infection, or bone tumor resection, the foot and ankle surgeon must be knowledgeable about current bone grafting options to make informed decisions. Innovation and technologic advances have produced an impressive and exciting array of options, advancing us closer to mimicking the gold standard: autograft. However, the sheer volume of available products makes it challenging for the foot and ankle surgeon to stay abreast of current bone graft technology. The purpose of this article is to simplify and classify current bone grafting options, discuss advantages and disadvantages, and provide relevant clinical examples.

During the last few decades, electrical current stimulation has gone from an investigational modality to an accepted method of treatment to assist with bone healing. This article provides an overview of electrical bone stimulation for nonunions in the foot and ankle.

Since its introduction into the market, negative pressure wound therapy (NPWT), also known as topical negative pressure, has become an important adjuvant therapy for the treatment of many types of wounds. Surgeons and physicians of all subspecialties have adopted NPWT into their practices. NPWT has become a mainstay in the management of lower extremity soft tissue pathology, especially in patients with traumatic, diabetic, postsurgical, and peripheral vascular disease-associated wounds. This article reviews the background, currently understood mechanisms of action, applications, contraindications, reported complications, advantages, criticisms, and techniques in the lower extremity.

Current Concepts and Techniques in Foot and Ankle Surgery

The goal of biologic resurfacing is to provide a smooth joint surface with a low coefficient of friction, which allows the joint to function with near normal biomechanics, as well as provide intermittent pressure, to the subchondral and cancellous bone. This unique combination often results in the formation of a "neocartilage-like" structure that can reduce pain and restore biomechanics. As well as giving a brief history of cutis arthroplasty, this article describes cases in which the ankle and first metatarsophalangeal joint underwent biologic resurfacing, with a 2-year postoperative follow up.

The Achilles tendon is the thickest and strongest tendon in the human body. In spite of this, it is also one of the most frequently ruptured tendons. This article reviews the history of and debate about the appropriate course of treatment. A case study of an Achilles repair illustrates that the use soft tissue matrices is a successful adjunct to both the primary repair and gastrocnemius recession, with full return to activity and no inflammatory response at long-term follow up. The authors anticipate that the use of soft tissue matrices for the repair of tendon and soft tissue defects will expand over time as this material has distinct advantages over synthetics and highly crosslinked biologic materials.

FORTHCOMING ISSUES

January 2010
The Pediatric Pes Planovalgus Deformity
Neal M. Blitz, DPM, *Guest Editor*

April 2010
The Rheumatoid Foot and Ankle
Lawrence A. DiDomenico, DPM,
Guest Editor

July 2010
Heel Pathology
George F. Wallace, DPM, *Guest Editor*

RECENT ISSUES

July 2009
The Importance of the First Ray
Lawrence A. Ford, DPM, FACFAS,
Guest Editor

April 2009
Update on Ankle Arthritis
Alan R. Catanzariti, DPM, FACFAS and
Robert W. Mendicino, DPM, FACFAS,
Guest Editors

January 2009
Revisional Foot and Ankle Surgery
Jerome K. Steck, DPM, FACFAS,
Guest Editor

RELATED INTEREST

Foot and Ankle Clinics
Volume 14, Issue 2, Pages 135–368 (June 2009)
Complex Injuries of the Foot and Ankle in Sport
Edited by D.A. Porter, MD, PhD

THE CLINICS ARE NOW AVAILABLE ONLINE!

Access your subscription at:
www.theclinics.com

Foreword

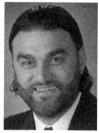

Thomas Zgonis, DPM, FACFAS
Consulting Editor

This issue focuses on the latest advancements, techniques, and innovations in wound and bone healing. A variety of topics covering the management of acute and chronic wounds and also bone fracture repair are described in detail. Recent advances in biotechnology and research in bioscaffolds, dermal replacements, orthobiologics, and bone stimulation have added a multitude of options to the surgeon's armamentarium. Dr. Landsman and his colleagues have done an extraordinary job of addressing the most beneficial changes in clinical management of recalcitrant wounds and bone healing. Particular emphasis is given to the soft tissue reconstruction of diabetic foot wounds and to the treatment of diabetic nonunions.

This issue also highlights my completion of one year as a Consulting Editor for the *Clinics in Podiatric Medicine and Surgery*. It has been a distinct honor to serve this outstanding role with a tremendous input of national and international editorial board members and contributing authors. I want to personally thank each one of you for your excellent contributions and publications. Finally, I hope that this issue will become a valuable tool and also provide you with great guidance when dealing with nonhealing wounds and nonunions.

Thomas Zgonis, DPM, FACFAS
Associate Professor and Chief
Division of Podiatric Medicine and Surgery
Department of Orthopaedic Surgery
University of Texas Health Science Center San Antonio
7703 Floyd Curl Drive - MSC 7776
San Antonio, TX 78229, USA

E-mail address:
zgonis@uthscsa.edu (T. Zgonis)

Clin Podiatr Med Surg 26 (2009) xi
doi:10.1016/j.cpm.2009.08.010
0891-8422/09/$ – see front matter © 2009 Elsevier Inc. All rights reserved.

Preface

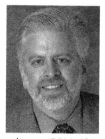

Adam Landsman, DPM, PhD, FACFAS
Guest Editor

Since the late 1700s, when John Hunter, MD, began his scientific assessment of human anatomy, and applied these principles to understanding human development and function, physicians have looked for better ways to make wounds heal and stimulate the growth of bone.[1] The science of getting bones to heal is still in its early stages, although the last 2 decades have shown us that the process is not only an active one, but potentially, one that can be controlled. The discovery of the piezoelectric effect and the generation of charges in bone placed under mechanical loads was a major breakthrough in its day.[2] Subsequently, this led to the pioneering work of Bassett and colleagues.[3] Who discovered that electrical fields can actually be created and used to trigger an ionic response in bone to stimulate proliferation. From there, refinement of stimulation protocols and improved understanding of how bones respond to charged stimulation led to the use of magnetic fields to trigger bone growth.

While a revolution was going on at the microscopic level, advances in fracture management also occurred. Plaster casts progressed to external fixation. Internal fixation moved in to the forefront, as the available materials for metal implants and screws improved, becoming less susceptible to corrosion. This led to the development of ambulatory surgery, where a bone could be repaired internally, and loaded almost immediately.

As time went by, we learned that bone healing could be controlled by applying mechanical loads. Very rigid internal fixation devices led to stress shielding and bone atrophy. This led to the development of absorbable fixation devices, which would do their job and then gradually disappear. Perhaps the most fascinating development in bone healing came from a small hospital in Siberia, where Ilizarov and associates[4] quietly pushed the boundaries with external fixation to create a completely new approach to deformity with their callous distraction technique.

Today, the research continues with the development of new ways to make manmade and natural products interact more efficiently. Implants now have special surface geometries to help the bone adhere more securely. Sintering and other techniques make bony ingrowth to the implants possible. The firm attachment between bone and manmade devices helped to spawn a whole new generation of ankle joint prostheses, retrograde nails, and new screws.

Clin Podiatr Med Surg 26 (2009) xiii–xv
doi:10.1016/j.cpm.2009.08.013
0891-8422/09/$ – see front matter © 2009 Elsevier Inc. All rights reserved.

podiatric.theclinics.com

Today, there is a renewed emphasis on getting bones to heal through biochemical stimulation. Recent advances have allowed scientists to isolate bone morphogenic proteins, in order to enhance their delivery at the site of bone healing. This has led to a variety of new products, and advancements in the preparation of new bone graft and bone graft substitutes. The new wave of products enhances bone growth and stimulates faster incorporation and integration into areas of need. The addition of these new tools helps the surgeon to fill and bridge defects, and trigger angiogenesis. When used in conjunction with various fixation devices, it creates new opportunities that have not been previously available.

Enhanced bone growth is only one chapter in the struggle to get tissues to heal. Soft tissue collagen bioscaffolds have now also become available to enhance the healing process. Collagen bioscaffolds provide the necessary structural components to facilitate soft tissue repair. These are acellular soft tissue matrices, fabricated from a variety of donor tissues such as human, bovine, and porcine skin, and intestinal mucosa. These materials contribute collagen, and are capable of stimulating angiogenesis, chemotaxis, and mitogenesis in native recipient tissues. New applications include reinforcement of ruptured ligaments and tendons, and may be useful as interpositional joint grafts in degenerated joints. Initially, reports in the literature implied that the stiffness and strength might be too low to augment the strength of soft tissue repairs. However, new data demonstrates that if properly prestressed, the strength of these collagen bioscaffolds may approach the strength of native tissues. Several physicians have reported great successes with this technique.

Wound healing is another area where advanced biologics have found a place. The first major breakthrough was the delivery of living cells prepared in the laboratory to the surface of difficult wounds. These living cell implants are capable of releasing growth factors to help with the healing process. However, in some cases, the slowly healing wound is in need of collagen matrix, rather than living cells, to advance the healing process. In these cases, collagen bioscaffolds fill a critical need. This scenario is especially common when wounds are treated with negative pressure wound therapy (NPWT). NPWT has proven to be a powerful tool for stimulating the formation of granulation tissue, but can leave the patient with a stagnant wound unless the highly vascular tissue is stabilized with collagen. In this case, the synergy achieved with NPWT and collagen bioscaffolds has led to some impressive results with difficult wounds.

Prevention of wounds is another area where collagen bioscaffolds may serve an important role. There have been many attempts to augment soft tissues susceptible to ulcerations, such as on the plantar surface of the foot. The historic work of Balkin[5] spanned over 40 years of research with silicone injections. Ultimately, he demonstrated that silicone could be used to temporarily relieve pain and dissipate focal pressures that could lead to ulcerations. However, concerns over injection of nonencapsulated liquid silicone ultimately led doctors to abandon this technique in favor of more natural products. Borrowing from the cosmetic surgeons, injections of hyaluronic acid and morselized collagen is in its infancy but appears to hold promise as a temporary solution. More recently, surgical procedures have been developed to implant collagen sheets that can be stitched in position, and will not migrate over time.

In this issue of the *Clinics in Podiatric Medicine and Surgery*, we have the opportunity to look at a variety of advanced biologic materials, and see how they can be used in different settings. We look at the differences and similarities associated with the various forms of collagen bioscaffolds from a histologic perspective. We also consider how these materials can be used in the reconstruction of soft tissues, including applications for ligament and tendon repair, joint resurfacing, and for augmentation of the plantar surface of the foot. There is a detailed description of newest bone graft materials—the authors describe some of the newest hybrid materials that have been enhanced to stimulate growth and incorporation. It is my sincere hope that the materials discussed in this issue will help the reader to identify new applications for these advanced biologics.

Adam Landsman, DPM, PhD, FACFAS
Assistant Professor of Surgery
Harvard Medical School
Attending Physician and Co-Director of Fellowship Training
Division of Podiatric Surgery
Beth Israel Deaconess Medical Center
1 Deaconess Road
Boston, MA 02215, USA

E-mail address:
alandsma@bidmc.harvard.edu (A. Landsman)

REFERENCES

1. Moore W. The knife man: the extraordinary life and times of John Hunter, father of modern surgery. 1st edition. New York: Broadway Pub; 2005.
2. Bassett CA, Becker RO. Generation of electric potentials by bone in response to mechanical stress. Science 1962;137:1063–4.
3. Bassett CA, Pawluk RJ, Pilla AA. Acceleration of fracture repair by electromagnetic fields. A surgically noninvasive method. Ann N Y Acad Sci 1974;238:242–62.
4. Ilizarov GA, Deviatov AA. [Surgical lengthening of the shin with simultaneous correction of deformities]. Ortop Travmatol Protez 1969;30(3):32–7 [in Russian].
5. Balkin SW. Injectable silicone and the foot: a 41-year clinical and histologic history. Dermatol Surg 2005;31(11 Pt 2):1555–9 [discussion: 1560].

Extracellular Matrix Biomaterials for Soft Tissue Repair

Kevin G. Cornwell, PhD[a], Adam Landsman, DPM, PhD, FACFAS[b],
Kenneth S. James, PhD[a],*

KEYWORDS

- Collagen • Extracellular matrix • Soft tissue reconstruction
- Bioscaffold • Acellular matrix • gTissue

The biological and physical augmentation provided by extracellular matrix (ECM) derived implants continues to challenge and refine the conventional wisdom of biomaterials. Human autograft and allograft ECM devices (eg, tendons, fascia, dermis, and ligaments) have been followed by bovine, porcine, and equine implants whose origins include heart valves, dermis, pericardium, and components of the intestine. Although artificial chemical crosslinking was initially thought necessary to limit the foreign body reaction to an implanted animal tissue and preserve implant integrity, it is now appreciated that different tissue-processing methodologies can produce xenogenic ECM devices with characteristic post-implantation responses ranging from the classic foreign body encapsulation of a permanent implant to one where the implant is degraded and resorbed to one where the processed ECM implant is populated by local fibroblasts and supporting vasculature to generate a new, metabolically active tissue.

ECM biomaterial technologies offer a range of device physicomechanical properties that can elicit distinct, biological responses after implantation. Reference to this class of implants as "acellular matrices" or "collagen scaffolds" can be a disservice, if the specifics of the devices and the possible impact on outcomes are not well understood. This article reviews the multiple ECM devices available for podiatric applications and highlights the impact of tissue source and processing on physicomechanical properties and host-implant interactions, with regard to surgical applications and clinical considerations.

[a] TEI Biosciences Inc., 7 Elkins Street, Boston, MA 02127, USA
[b] Division of Podiatric Surgery, Beth Israel Deaconess Medical Center, 1 Deaconess Road, MA 02215, USA
* Corresponding author.
E-mail address: kjames@teibio.com (K.S. James).

Clin Podiatr Med Surg 26 (2009) 507–523
doi:10.1016/j.cpm.2009.08.001
0891-8422/09/$ – see front matter
© 2009 Elsevier Inc. All rights reserved.
podiatric.theclinics.com

PRODUCT PROCESSING AND COMPOSITION

The composition of an ECM biomaterial reflects the original constituents of the source tissue and the selected processing methodology that may act to preserve, remove, or modify various components of the source tissue.

Tissue Source (Material Origin)

All ECM-based implants are derived from mammalian tissues, including dermis, pericardium, and small intestinal submucosa (SIS), although other processed tissues may enter the market in the future. These tissues are harvested at different developmental stages from various species, including human, porcine, equine, and bovine in ages ranging from fetal to adult (**Table 1**). Although the ECM of each, regardless of species, is composed primarily of fibrillar collagens, inherent source variation (tissue, species, and age) manifests in the form of different

- Microstructure
- Specific composition including the
  - o Quantities and types of noncollagenous proteins, glycosaminoglycans (GAGs), or other factors
  - o Ratios of collagens (Types I, III, IV)
- Mechanical properties
- Physical dimensions including available final product sizes and/or thickness

An example of the diversity in ECM microstructure as a function of tissue type and species is highlighted in **Fig. 1**. Dermis ECM is discernible by the crosshatch pattern of woven collagen fibers in contrast to the thin, laminated layers of intestinal submucosa that constitute SIS-based ECM biomaterials. The microstructure can also vary by age and location of harvest. As a calf develops through fetal stages into adulthood, the thickness of the dermis increases and the collagen fibers and cables that make up the dermal architecture grow in diameter. The biochemical composition of the ECM can also change with age. For example, fetal and neonatal dermis has between 3 and 5 times more Type III collagen than adult dermis,[1–3] Type III collagen is a form of fibrillar collagen associated with healing and developing tissues.[4–6] The choice of tissue source also determines the possible width and breadth of the final product, based on the ability to harvest large pieces of uniform, continuous material.

Processing

Although the original source tissue dictates the characteristics of the device, the processing conditions under which an ECM biomaterial is prepared can equally influence characteristics of the final product. Many of the numerous materials available for clinical consideration are processed in different, often proprietary, ways. Although the specifics of the chemical or enzymatic steps and washes often remain unknown, the original goals and results can be described. Some ECM biomaterials are processed to remove cells but to retain most other ECM components. For example, GraftJacket (Wright Medical Technology, Arlington, TN) is a minimally processed allograft derived from human dermis and reported to retain noncollagenous components of the ECM including elastin and proteoglycans.[7,8] Restore (DePuy, Warsaw, IN, USA) and Surgisis (Cook, Bloomington, IN, USA) are SIS-based materials that have been reported to retain fibronectin (FGF-2) and GAGs, but not vascular endothelial growth factor (VEGF).[9,10] Alternatively, fetal bovine dermis biomaterials (SurgiMend and PriMatrix, TEI Biosciences, Boston, MA, USA; TissueMend, Stryker Orthopedics, Kalamazoo, MI, USA), have been processed using a method originally intended as

Table 1
Overview of the diverse set of clinically available ECM biomaterials by tissue source, manufacturer, specifications, and applications

Trade Name	Animal Source	Tissue Source	Cross-linker	Terminal Sterilization	Thickness*	Cleared Indications**	Marketer	Manufacturer
TissueMend	Fetal Bovine		None	Low Temperature Ethylene Oxide	~1 mm	Tendon reinforcement	Stryker Orthopaedics	TEI Biosciences
SurgiMend	Neonatal Bovine		None	Low Temperature Ethylene Oxide	~2, 3, or 4 mm	Hernia repair / Plastic & reconstructive surgery	TEI Biosciences	TEI Biosciences
SurgiMend 2.0, 3.0, 4.0	Neonatal Bovine		None	Low Temperature Ethylene Oxide	~2, 3, or 4 mm	Hernia repair / Plastic & reconstructive surgery	TEI Biosciences	TEI Biosciences
PriMatrix	Fetal Bovine		None	Low Temperature Ethylene Oxide	~1 mm	Skin and wound healing	TEI Biosciences	TEI Biosciences
Permacol	Adult Porcine	Dermis	HMDI	Gamma Irradiation	0.5 - 1.5 mm	Hernia repair / Plastic & reconstructive surgery	Covidien	Tissue Science Laboratories (Covidien)
Zimmer Collagen Patch	Adult Porcine	Dermis	HMDI	Gamma Irradiation	1.5 mm	Tendon reinforcement	Zimmer	Tissue Science Laboratories (Covidien)
CollaMend	Adult Porcine	Dermis	EDC	Ethylene Oxide	0.8 - 1.2 mm	Hernia repair / Plastic & reconstructive surgery	Davol (Bard)	Davol (Bard)
Conexa	Adult Porcine	Dermis	None	E-beam	1.5 - 2.0 mm	Tendon reinforcement	Tornier	Lifecell (KCI)
Strattice	Adult Porcine	Dermis	None	None	0.8 - 3.3 mm	Hernia repair		Lifecell (KCI)
Alloderm	Adult Human	Dermis	None	None	0.5 - 2.0 mm	By US law, tissue transplants intended only for homologous use		Lifecell (KCI)
GraftJacket	Adult Human	Dermis	None	None	0.4 - 4 mm	By US law, tissue transplants intended only for homologous use	Wright Medical	Lifecell (KCI)
FlexHD	Adult Human	Dermis	None	None		By US law, tissue transplants intended only for homologous use	Ethicon (J&J)	Musculoskeletal Transplant Foundation
AlloPatch	Adult Human	Dermis	None	None		By US law, tissue transplants intended only for homologous use	Musculoskeletal Transplant Foundation	Musculoskeletal Transplant Foundation
AlloMax	Adult Human	Dermis	None	Gamma Irradiation		By US law, tissue transplants intended only for homologous use	Davol (Bard)	RTI Biologics
NeoForm	Adult Human	Dermis	None	Gamma Irradiation	0.8 - 1.8	By US law, tissue transplants intended only for homologous use	Mentor	RTI Biologics
Restore	Adult Porcine	Small Intestinal Submucosa (SIS)	None	E-Beam Radiation	0.3 - 1.0 mm	Tendon reinforcement	DePuy	DePuy
Surgisis Biodesign	Adult Porcine	Small Intestinal Submucosa (SIS)	None	Ethylene Oxide	0.3 - 1.0 mm	Reconstructive surgery / Hernia repair	Cook	Cook
Oasis	Adult Porcine	Small Intestinal Submucosa (SIS)	None	Ethylene Oxide	~0.1 mm	Skin and wound healing	Healthpoint	Cook
CuffPatch	Adult Porcine	Small Intestinal Submucosa (SIS)	EDC	Gamma Irradiation	~1 mm	Tendon reinforcement	Biomet/Organogenesis	Organogenesis
OrthAdapt	Adult Equine	Pericardium	EDC		0.5 - 1.2 mm	Hernia repair / Tendon reinforcement	Organogenesis	(formerly Pegasus Biologics, acq. in 2009)
Unite	Adult Equine	Pericardium	EDC		0.5 - 1.2 mm	Skin and wound healing	Organogenesis	(formerly Pegasus Biologics, acq. in 2009)
Veritas	Adult Bovine	Pericardium	None	E-Beam Radiation	0.3 - 0.6 mm	Hernia repair / Muscle flap reinforcement		Synovis
Peri-Strips	Adult Bovine	Pericardium	None	E-Beam Radiation	0.2 - 1.2 mm	Staple-line reinforcement		Synovis

*Total range of product thickness, but versions may be sold with tighter range subsets
**see Instructions For Use for individual products for detailed and complete indications.

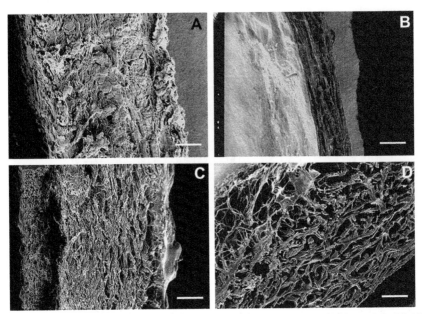

Fig. 1. Scanning electron micrographs of cross-sections of (*A*) Permacol, (*B*) Surgisis, (*C*) Alloderm, and (*D*) SurgiMend. The woven collagen fiber architecture of porcine dermis (*A*) is similar to that of human dermis (*C*) and bovine dermis (*D*), and the thin laminated layers of SIS (*B*) are apparent. Differences in the porosity of the 3 dermis-based tissues and SIS are also apparent. (Scale bar = 200 μm).

a matrix preservation technique for scientific investigations of the collagen fiber architecture[11] where all lipids, fats, carbohydrates, and noncollagenous proteins are removed. Thus the composition of this material is primarily Type I and Type III collagen, conserved in a native and undamaged state. Final device manufacturing steps for some products include lyophilization or solvent evaporation to remove water before sterilization, and others are sold in their final rinse solution. Materials that are dried or lyophilized can be shipped and stored dry for extended periods. Using lyophilization, the pore size (see **Fig. 1**), rehydration rate, and ability of blood and cells to penetrate the matrix can be modulated.

Processing: Artificial Crosslinking

"Crosslinking" is a term borrowed from polymer chemistry that describes chemical bonds between polymer chains. The collagen fiber architecture of the ECM is a polymer network, and over time a natural mechanism to stabilize the fiber matrix through intermolecular bonds by lysyl oxidase has evolved.[12] Historically, artificial crosslinking was first employed to mask the antigenic response of xenograft heart valves using gluteraldehyde. Subsequent scientific investigations into this and other similar methods determined that crosslinking chemistry could be used to stabilize artificially collagen materials reconstituted from homogenized sources, reducing the otherwise rapid degradation of these biomaterials in vivo.[12] More recently, some ECM biomaterials have adopted these different chemical crosslinking methodologies to achieve intended effects by altering cell-matrix interactions and mechanical properties. For example, Permacol (Coviden, Mansfield, MA) is crosslinked with hexamethylene diisocyanate (HMDI) to make a permanent collagen implant, hence the titular conjunction. Others have used 1-ethyl-3-(3-dimethylaminopropyl) carbodiimide (EDC), because of its ability to add crosslinks without retaining the crosslinking molecule,[13] while surreptitiously being investigated as a conjugation method for adding other desirable molecules and growth factors that could be incorporated into future devices. As a result, addition of these nonnative crosslinks alters the host response at a cellular level. One resulting change is a decrease in the susceptibility of the collagen molecule to enzymatic degradation, namely by matrix metalloproteinases (MMPs),[14,15] thereby increasing in vivo persistence. However, these artificial modifications can also affect growth factor binding to collagen, cell attachment, and migration,[16,17] and lead to recognition as a foreign body by the host (see section on Host-implant interactions later in this article). Many ECM biomaterials are now not intentionally crosslinked, as new processing methodologies have achieved clinically acceptable persistence without the need for artificial stabilization.

Processing: Sterilization

Most ECM biomaterials are terminally sterilized to ensure that the final product has no infectious bacteria or viruses. These methods include the use of ethylene oxide (EO) gas, gamma irradiation, or electron-beam (e-beam) irradiation. EO sterilization requires a porous and dry final product to allow the gas into and exhaust out of the matrix; irradiation need not be dry, but may crosslink or denature the final product.[18–21] Allografts are the exception, as most are aseptically processed and treated with antibiotics.

Product Processing and Composition: Summary

In summary, ECM biomaterial processing varies between soft tissue substitutes. Different chemical washes and rinses are used in processing and manufacturing; some are crosslinked; some are dried or lyophilized; a variety of sterilizing methodologies are used. Any or all of these steps can alter the composition of the resulting ECM biomaterial. The individual parameters of the same methods may differ among products. For example, freezing times and temperatures during lyophilization can alter ice-crystal formation, resulting in different size crystals, and subsequent material porosity. Differences must be evaluated by investigating the final product composition, physical/mechanical properties, and the host-implant interactions.

PHYSICAL-MECHANICAL PROPERTIES

The physical and mechanical properties of an ECM biomaterial are a function of the tissue source, processing, crosslinking, and sterilization. The physical dimensions of the device can be strongly correlated with those of the source material. For example, the size of the tissue available for harvest from the host determines the sizes available for processing into final product. Currently, Permacol and SurgiMend, derived from porcine and bovine dermis, respectively, are available in sheets up to 25 by 40 cm, while most human autografts are limited to smaller sizes related to the ability to harvest tissue using dermatomes. Within this subset of dermal ECM biomaterials, the thickness can range from approximately 0.5 mm to 4 mm, although most products are available in an average thickness of 1 mm. In contrast, SIS devices are typically thin; the thickest, 10-layer laminated version of Surgisis is less than 1 mm thick on average.

The initial mechanical properties of ECM biomaterials have been widely investigated,[22–25] and are dictated by the microstructure of the material. Thicker materials have an increased load-carrying capacity, and the properties of any ECM biomaterial can be altered with chemical crosslinking methodologies. However, the stress-strain characteristics of acellular dermal materials are similar to those of the native tissue from which they were derived (**Fig. 2**). As a result of comparing elastic modulus measurements (taken without prestretching and in the low modulus region) with native tendon, some studies have suggested that these materials "may not be capable of providing appreciable mechanical reinforcement" to tendon repair.[26] Although these data can be refuted when ECM biomaterials are tested in clinically relevant models,[22,27] the goal in using the materials stems from their ability to reinforce without the conventional stress-shielding or material property mismatch problems associated with synthetics that are orders of magnitude stiffer than native tendon. In addition, these studies of initial mechanical properties ignore that the properties of the implanted ECM biomaterial change with time, making the initial mechanical strength a poor indicator of ultimate clinical success.

HOST-IMPLANT INTERACTIONS

Conventional wound healing is a highly coordinated cellular response to injury, reviewed in other studies specifically for skin[28,29] and tendon.[30,31] Normal wound healing following surgical intervention results in limited acute inflammation lasting approximately 2 weeks, followed by a remodeling phase lasting from weeks to years, as the repaired tissue is slowly reorganized. How the addition of an ECM biomaterial affects this process, and conversely, how this process affects the implanted device, can vary within this subset of products. A limited number of comparative studies or clinical trials are available for many devices. However, for some products there is a solid foundation of literature and experience that identifies at least five possible biological responses, including:

- ECM nonincorporating responses
  - (1) Encapsulation
  - (2) Rejection
- ECM incorporating responses
  - (3) Resorption
  - (4) Integration with progressive degradation
  - (5) Adoption and adaptation

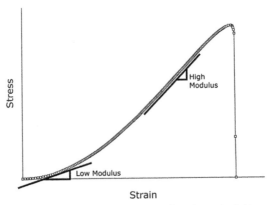

Fig. 2. Characteristic stress-strain curve for SurgiMend under uniaxial tension. An initial low modulus region, a function of collagen fiber reorientation and alignment, is followed by a linear high modulus region.

Nonincorporating

Encapsulation

The subset of host-implant interactions most familiar to those accustomed to using polymer meshes or sutures is crosslinked materials. The acute and chronic inflammatory profile of Permacol, HMDI crosslinked porcine dermis, is consistent with that of the classic foreign body response to nonresorbable biomaterials ending without incorporation, but rather in fibrous encapsulation.[32,33] Initially the response includes a heavy collection of macrophages and neutrophils at the periphery of the implant (**Fig. 3**G, I). With time, macrophages fuse together to form foreign body giant cells as the host attempts to wall off the foreign object with a layer of dense connective tissue, that is, fibrous encapsulation (see **Fig. 3**J). In a study compared with Permacol, the reported response to Collamend (Davol, Warwick, RI, USA), an EDC crosslinked porcine dermis product, found similar results between the two materials, including moderate chronic inflammation, limited to the periphery of the implant at 6 months with no cellular or vascular infiltration.[7] This response can be desirable if the expected clinical outcomes are congruous with those typified by nondegradable polymers or metals, used in many products, including hip implants and surgical meshes. However, encapsulated ECM biomaterials can be prone to many of the same complications as other permanent implants that react following the classic foreign body response,[34] such as migration or transcutaneous extrusion.[33,35]

Rejection

Other interactions have been described for crosslinked ECM biomaterials that deviate from the permanent implant, foreign body response. For example, CuffPatch (Organogenesis, Canton, MA, USA), an EDC crosslinked SIS patch indicated for tendon repair, initially demonstrated a host response similar to other crosslinked ECM biomaterials, marked by "a dense accumulation of neutrophils and mononuclear cells located primarily at the edge of the implanted device" at 1 week (see **Fig. 3**G) without cell infiltration into the matrix. However, by 16 weeks, the CuffPatch was partially degraded with a "robust inflammatory cell reaction and multinucleated giant cells throughout the matrix" (see **Fig. 3**H). In this case, the host response was more successful in rejecting and deconstructing the foreign body as indicated by strong chronic inflammation, giant cell accumulation in and around the matrix, and degradation.[36]

Incorporating

For devices that can be incorporated, a fundamentally different set of host-implant interactions occur. (Incorporation is a term often used in the discussion of ECM biomaterials clinically and in the literature, but without clear definition. From the authors' experience, most questions regarding ECM biomaterial incorporation are related to whether the material will allow cells and blood vessels to penetrate the matrix. Therefore, in this article incorporation is defined as the ability of an ECM biomaterial to repopulate with host cells and revascularize with host blood vessels.) Initially, cells can penetrate and populate these matrices, and produce proteins and enzymes to simultaneously break down collagen fibers and reassemble collagen fibers to replace the tissue. The rate of breakdown and assembly have not been accurately quantified for any of these materials. Ultimately the rate can be considered dependent on the multitude of variables between products such as the retained ECM components following processing to remove cells, the sterilization type, and the starting structure of the fibrous network making up the anatomic location of harvest (ie, pericardium, dermis, intestinal submucosa).

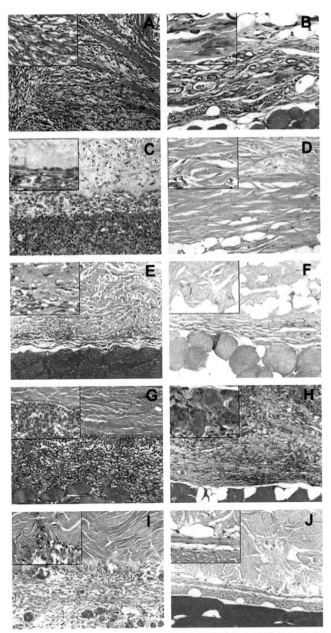

Fig. 3. Histology of ECM biomaterials implanted on a 1-cm² partial thickness muscle defect in rats at 1 week (*left*) and 16 weeks (*right*). Restore (porcine SIS) was infiltrated with a large quantity of inflammatory cells degrading and separating the layers of the device (*A*) and no evidence of the device was seen at 16 weeks (*B*). Dense populations of mononuclear inflammatory cells were seen at the edges of Alloderm (human dermis) (*C*) and the implant was partially degraded by 16 weeks (*D*). The SurgiMend (fetal bovine dermis) was repopulated with host cells with minimal inflammatory response (*E*) and "remained virtually unchanged from the time of implantation" at 16 weeks (*F*). A dense accumulation of neutrophils and mononuclear cells was found at the edge of the CuffPatch (crosslinked SIS) early (*G*) with chronic inflammation and foreign body giant cells present later (*H*). Early accumulation of neutrophils, mononuclear cells, and foreign body giant cells at the periphery of Permacol (crosslinked porcine dermis) was present early (*I*) and there was almost no evidence of scaffold degradation at 16 weeks (*J*). (*From* Valentin JE, Badylak JS, et al. Extracellular matrix bioscaffolds for orthopaedic applications. A comparative histologic study. J Bone Joint Surg Am 2006;88(12):2673–86; with permission.)

Resorption

At the other end of the device-host biological response spectrum, ECM biomaterials are available that can be rapidly resorbed by the host. Derived from multilaminated layers of thin intestinal submucosa (non–crosslinked SIS technology), Restore and Surgisis retain certain noncollagenous components of the ECM that have been demonstrated to alter cellular interactions. For example, these materials have been reported to retain FGF-2 and GAGs, but not VEGF.[9,10] In studies, these materials were rapidly infiltrated by inflammatory cells after as little as 7 days (see **Fig. 3**A). Cells separate the layers of the laminated collagen material, leading to rapid resorption of the material and replacement with disorganized scar tissue (see **Fig. 3**B). Similarly, SIS materials have been described as rapidly degraded in a canine model,[37] rapidly resorbed in an ovine tendon augmentation study,[38] and delaminate by intense infiltration with polymorphonuclear, mononuclear, and foreign body giant cells in primate body wall repair.[7] The typical expected result following implantation of these devices is rapid degradation and resorption, resulting in scar tissue formation.[7] Whether this strong response is purely inflammatory or can be more readily associated with immunologic rejection common to cellular xenografts is still being debated. Stronger than expected clinical signs of inflammation have been witnessed clinically in humans[39,40] with multiple hypothetical explanations related to the processing of SIS materials and constituents retained in the matrix. Some reports found SIS materials containing remnant cell nuclei and other cellular debris that could be immunogenic.[40] Others have investigated the presence of the immunogenic epitope alpha-Gal retained in SIS materials.[7] The alpha-Gal epitope is found abundantly expressed on glycoconjugates of nonprimate mammals[41] and associated with xenograft rejection considering an estimated 1% of circulating human immunoglobulin (IgG) is anti-Gal.[41,42] The presence of anti-Gal antibodies in histological slides of preimplant SIS[7] and anti-Gal antibodies in patients with SIS implants have been reported.[43] Regardless of the immunogenic potential of SIS biomaterials, processing that retains noncollagenous proteins, growth factors, and GAGs[9,10] may promote the strong inflammatory profile, particularly if these retained constituents have been damaged during processing.

Integration with progressive degradation

Another example of a different expected biological response with a non–crosslinked ECM biomaterial is that of GraftJacket. Graftjacket (Alloderm), sold as an allograft and derived from human dermis, is minimally processed and reported to retain noncollagenous components of the ECM, including elastin and proteoglycans.[7,8] Alloderm is incorporated, including repopulation with host cells and vasculature.[8] The early inflammatory response at 7 days is marked by dense layers of mononuclear cells at the periphery of the device (see **Fig. 3**C). These cells, likely a combination of neutrophils and macrophages among others, surround the device and penetrate the outer layers of the implant (see **Fig. 3**C). This low-grade inflammation persists in parts of the matrix, typically in the outer regions, and the implant is slowly degraded.[44] In a subcutaneous implant study in rats, a human acellular dermis implant is evaluated at 1, 4, 8, and 12 weeks after implantation (**Fig. 4**).[44] These researchers describe a marked decrease in volume, including a decrease greater than 60% in implant dimension, whereby "host cell infiltration and neovascularization occurred only around the implant."[44] The material is slowly degraded from the periphery toward the center of the implant and partially replaced with fibrous connective tissue. Animal and human studies report a similar phenomenon as thinning to translucence in rat studies[45] and clinical failure in human studies.[46,47]

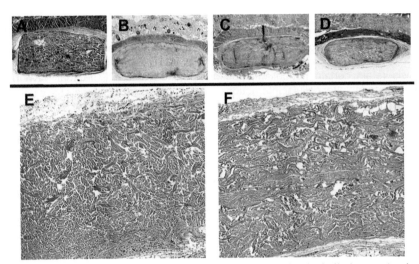

Fig. 4. Histology images of subcutaneous histological sections (*top*) of Alloderm stained with Masson trichrome and subcutaneously implanted in rats demonstrate slow steady degradation of the implant from the periphery toward the center with time progression between (*A*) 1, (*B*) 4, (*C*) 8, and (*D*) 12 weeks. Sections of SurgiMend (*bottom*) stained with hematoxylin and eosin (H&E) and implanted subcutaneously in rats show the ECM biomaterial populated by host cells at 4 weeks (*E*) and persisting without apparent alteration in the cell density or larger collagen fiber architecture for 15 months (*F*) in this non–load-bearing application. (*Images A–D courtesy of* Hwang K, Hwang JH, et al. Experimental study of autologous cartilage, acellular cadaveric dermis, lyophilized bovine pericardium, and irradiated bovine tendon: applicability to nasal tip plasty. J Craniofac Surg 2007;18(3):551–8; with permission.)

Adoption and adaptation

Encapsulation and degradation are not the only results in the use of ECM biomaterials. Non–crosslinked ECM biomaterials derived from fetal bovine dermis (for example SurgiMend or TissueMend) demonstrate adoption by host fibroblasts, and can persist as a new, generative tissue (gTissue), being adapted as necessary to meet the demands of the mechanical loading environment. At the time of implantation, the highly porous material readily traps blood, acting as a sponge to trap cells, growth factors, and cytokines, to seed the matrix. The biomaterial is rapidly repopulated with host cells and supporting vasculature. Acute histology indicates a muted inflammatory response in comparison with other ECM biomaterials (see **Fig. 3**E, F), including sparse quantities of neutrophils, and macrophages. By 4 weeks, in a rat intramuscular implant, the material is populated with fibroblasts, and a few remaining inflammatory cells (**Fig. 5**A). In contrast to other ECM biomaterials, the interface between muscle and implant is essentially seamless and the collagen fiber architecture of the material appears essentially unchanged (see **Fig. 5**A). By 12 weeks, the intramuscular implant persists with no perceptible alteration to the collagen fiber structure and no chronic inflammatory response (see **Fig. 5**B). The material is still populated with host fibroblasts, and a few remaining apoptotic immune cells, including granulocytes and macrophages, can be found, typical of resolving wound healing. Fetal ECM biomaterials in subcutaneous non–load-bearing applications have been tested in rats after 15 months with the gTissue remaining as a living connective tissue, adopted by the host, populated with fibroblasts, without inflammation, change in cell quantity, or major alteration in the larger collagen fiber architecture (see **Fig. 4**F).

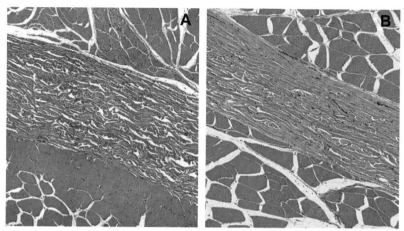

Fig. 5. H&E-stained sections of SurgiMend after (*A*) 4 weeks and (*B*) 12 weeks intramuscular implantation in rats. At both time points, the material had incorporated at the implant site, with no evidence of inflammation or fibrous encapsulation. The material was repopulated with host cells, particularly fibroblasts. The edge of the material on all sides was in direct contact with muscle without the classic signs of a foreign body response (ie, no accumulation of inflammatory cells at the implant periphery, no foreign giant cells, no fibrous encapsulation).

However, similar to native connective tissue, gTissue can be adapted by the host if the appropriate cell signalling exists. Although the precise set of signaling conditions modulating the fetal ECM biomaterial is undefined, some parameters have been identified. Clear differences are seen in external skin wounds compared with internal surgical placement (see section on Applications). Furthermore, the mechanical loading environment appears to be a controlling factor in fetal ECM biomaterial adaptation. For example, replacement of tendon in a small animal model resulted in the rapid adaptation of the collagen fiber architecture of the material from its characteristic crosshatch pattern to the more aligned and oriented fibrillar structure of native tendon in as little as 4 weeks after repair (**Fig. 6**).

APPLICATIONS

The use of ECM biomaterials is rapidly expanding as the general utility of these materials has gained acceptance. Understanding the clinical advantages and limitations of these materials is crucial to their overall effectiveness in aiding patient outcomes. Currently, only limited clinical data have been published describing the use of any individual material listed in **Table 1**, and none have been reported in direct comparison. Clinicians' goals and patient specific intended outcomes should be matched to the appropriate expected responses described above. Therefore, in the following discussion, cases familiar to the authors, and from the clinical experience of one author (A.L.), are highlighted in which the adoption and adaptation response, gTissue functionality, and lack of inflammation were desirable characteristics.

Tendon and Ligament Repair

ECM biomaterials have been used in tendon repair procedures for more than a decade with clinical success. These materials are used to augment primary repair of tendons, to reinforce weakness, and to promote healing in a tissue that represents a significant

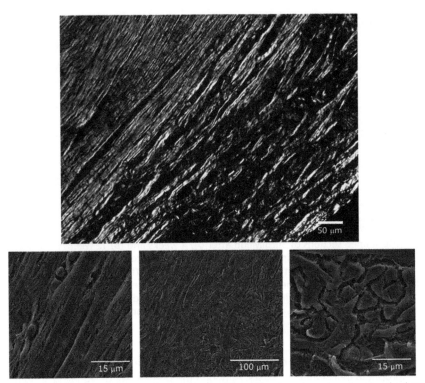

Fig. 6. Polarized light microscopy image (*top*) of SurgiMend undergoing structural adaptation in response to loading in a rat tendon repair application. The crosshatch pattern of the dermis-derived material can be seen on the right at 4 weeks post implantation in a tendon defect. SurgiMend on the left has been adapted to the loading environment and now has a collagen fiber architecture indicative of tendon. High magnification SEM images highlight the seamless transition region (*bottom middle*) and the collagen fiber orientation and alignment of the SurgiMend (*bottom right*) and the SurgiMend adapted into tendon (*bottom left*).

clinical challenge. Tendons tend to have a limited vascular supply, and large tears, like those common in the rotator cuff, do not heal spontaneously, necessitating surgical intervention with high recurrence rates. In podiatric applications, these materials are commonly used as a wrap during Achilles tendon repair, tendon-lengthening procedures, and other foot and ankle tendon reattachment procedures.[48–50] For example, SurgiMend has been successfully used to reinforce the repair of a complete rupture of the tibialis anterior tendon in a diabetic patient with results after 6 months demonstrating a return to full strength (grade increased from 2 to 4 out of 5 on the Medical Research Council scale of manual muscle strength) and restoration of heel-walking ability.[51] Other case studies have reported use of SurgiMend in the repair of an injured posterior tibiotalar ligament, in which the material was sutured under high tension (**Fig. 7**B). In these procedures, when primary attachment cannot be achieved and suture wire with bone anchors is required to reattach the torn ligament, SurgiMend has been used to promote biologic regeneration of tendon tissue around a supporting suture in what would otherwise be a large tissue gap.

Novel uses of these materials are redefining classic tendon repair by taking advantage of the unique attributes of certain ECM biomaterials. In one particular case study,

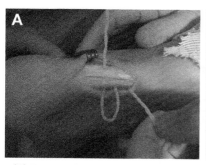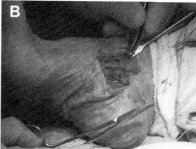

Fig. 7. (*A*) Reapproximation of an Achilles tendon after debridement of the central portion, weaving SurgiMend string. The patient reported less pain and a more rapid return to mobility. (*B*) SurgiMend sutured under high tension in the repair of an injured posterior tibiotalar ligament.

a thin string of SurgiMend, approximately 2 mm wide by 1.5 mm thick by 25 cm long, was used in the surgical repair of an Achilles tendon in a patient suffering from chronic Achilles tendonosis. After longitudinal debridement of the deteriorated, inflamed, central portion of the Achilles tendon, the tissue was reapproximated using the SurgiMend string rather than standard, nonresorbable suture (see **Fig. 7**A). Under these conditions, a material that can be adopted and adapted to the patient without inciting an inflammatory response is ideally suited, considering it is being applied in a disease state associated with excessive chronic inflammation. The results for this particular patient included a return to full weight-bearing activities in half the expected time and an almost immediate reduction in pain.

Plastic and Reconstructive Procedures of the Foot and Ankle

Surgeons are creatively expanding the repertoire of procedures that use these devices, particularly for plastic and reconstructive procedures. Our experience with SurgiMend alone has seen the product successfully used in plantar fat pad augmentation and resurfacing of the metatarsophalangeal (MTP) joint in lower limb procedures. In clinical use by the author (A.L.), SurgiMend has been demonstrated to support adipose tissue growth in the stabilization of the calcaneal fat pad. In patients with advance degenerative joint disease or hallux rigidus of the first MTP, SurgiMend has been wrapped around the bone and remaining cartilage following debridement of exostoses and damaged cartilage similar to the methodology employed by Berlet and colleagues.[52] This procedure has helped restore joint motion, reduce pain, and delay or eliminate the need for more complicated and nonreversible procedures like arthrodesis or joint replacement with a prothesis.

Skin and Wound Healing

In podiatric medicine, one of the most common applications for ECM biomaterials is in dermal regeneration and the healing of difficult open wounds, although the mechanism of healing and repair is not equivalent to that of surgical implantation. Closing complex full-thickness wounds of the foot and ankle is challenging because of the varying causes and underlying conditions leading to pressure ulcers, most notably diabetes. Ulcers may persist for months to years, and practicing podiatrists may try repeated applications and multiple products before finding the right means of achieving wound closure. ECM biomaterials have been demonstrated to improve

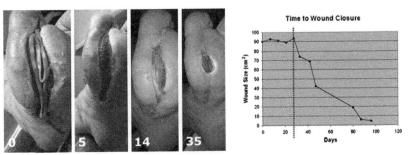

Fig. 8. The use of PriMatrix strips following infection of an ulceration below the first metatarsal head. After extensive debridement and essentially no progress toward closure by 4 weeks, PriMatrix strips were placed (time 28, dotted line on graph). Following the initial application, a second application was added 5 days later as the wound rapidly progressed toward eventual complete closure. (*Courtesy of* Landsman and colleagues, American College of Foot and Ankle Surgeons, Long Beach, CA, USA, February 2008.)

outcomes in the treatment of diabetic ulcers in prospective[53–55] and retrospective[56] clinical studies. For example, in a patient presenting with a long ulceration following infection below the metatarsal head on the left foot, 4 weeks of treatment with negative pressure wound therapy demonstrated essentially no progress toward closure, but immediately progressed toward closure following the application of PriMatrix, an ECM biomaterial similar to SurgiMend but indicated for skin wounds (**Fig. 8**). These materials are successful in promoting a vascular granulation tissue[57] even in particularly difficult wounds in high-risk diabetic patients with additional complicating factors such as peripheral artery disease, peripheral neuropathy, rheumatoid arthritis, and end-stage renal disease on dialysis.[58] Furthermore, these materials can be successful in building tissue in deep tunneling wounds and over exposed bone.

In the treatment of full thickness wounds, multiple applications of the ECM biomaterial may be required before full closure; on follow-up evaluation of the wound, the material can no longer be distinguished from the new granulation tissue. In contrast to the noted response to SurgiMend during surgical implantation, the mechanism of healing does not appear to follow the sequence of events whereby the material is repopulated with cells and persists. Difficulty in reproducing these complex wound-healing environments in nonclinical studies has left this area of investigation largely unstudied. However, the ability of non–crosslinked ECM biomaterials to be altered by the host, and to do so without inciting inflammation, are probable factors distinguishing this mechanism of healing.

SUMMARY

The many options and expanding utility of ECM biomaterials have encouraged clinicians to improve their knowledge of the use and application of these biomaterials. There are diverse biological responses when using different ECM biomaterials in different clinical situations. Although the degradation or encapsulation that can result from using some ECM biomaterials may be acceptable, tissue building may also be necessary, facilitated by appropriate selection and understanding of implant conditions. An understanding of the distinguishing characteristics of ECM biomaterials for intended outcomes can improve patient results and create new possibilities for the healing and repair of challenging foot and ankle conditions.

REFERENCES

1. Mays PK, Bishop JE, Laurent GJ. Age-related changes in the proportion of types I and III collagen. Mech Ageing Dev 1988;45:203–12.
2. Ramshaw J. Distribution of type III collagen in bovine skin of various ages. Connect Tissue Res 1986;14:307–14.
3. Smith LT, Holbrook KA, Madri JA. Collagen types I, III and V in human embryonic and fetal skin. Am J Anat 1986;175:507–21.
4. Barnes MJ, Morton LF, Bennett RC, et al. Presence of type III collagen in guinea-pig dermal scar. Biochem J 1976;157:263–6.
5. Haukipuro K, Melkko J, Risteli L, et al. Synthesis of type I collagen in healing wounds in humans. Ann Surg 1991;213(1):75–80.
6. Liu X, Wu H, Byrne M, et al. Type III collagen is crucial for collagen I fibrillogenesis and for normal cardiovascular development. Proc Natl Acad Sci U S A 1997;94(5):1852–6.
7. Sandor M, Xu H, Connor J, et al. Host response to implanted porcine-derived biologic materials in a primate model of abdominal wall repair. Tissue Eng Part A 2008;14(12):2021–31.
8. Wong AK, Schonmyer BH, Singh P, et al. Histologic analysis of angiogenesis and lymphangiogenesis in acellular human dermis. Plast Reconstr Surg 2008;121(4):1144–52.
9. Hodde J, Janis A, Ernst D, et al. Effects of sterilization on an extracellular matrix scaffold: part I. Composition and matrix architecture. J Mater Sci Mater Med 2007a;18(4):537–43.
10. Hodde J, Janis A, Hiles M. Effects of sterilization on an extracellular matrix scaffold: part II. Bioactivity and matrix interaction. J Mater Sci Mater Med 2007b;18(4):545–50.
11. Ohtani O, Ushiki T, Taguchi T, et al. Collagen fibrillar networks as skeletal frameworks: a demonstration by cell-maceration/scanning electron microscope method. Arch Histol Cytol 1988;51(3):249–61.
12. Friess W. Collagen – biomaterial for drug delivery. Eur J Pharm Biopharm 1998;45(2):113–36.
13. Wnek GE, Bowlin GL. Encyclopedia of biomaterials and biomedical engineering. New York: Marcel Dekker, Inc; 2004.
14. Charulatha V, Rajaram A. Influence of different crosslinking treatments on the physical properties of collagen membranes. Biomaterials 2003;24(5):759–67.
15. Weadock KS, Miller EJ, Keuffel EL, et al. Effect of physical crosslinking methods on collagen-fiber durability in proteolytic solutions. J Biomed Mater Res 1996;32(2):221–6.
16. Cornwell KG, Downing BR, Pins GD. Characterizing fibroblast migration on discrete collagen threads for applications in tissue regeneration. J Biomed Mater Res A 2004;71(1):55–62.
17. Cornwell KG, Lei P, Andreadis ST, et al. Crosslinking of discrete self-assembled collagen threads: effects on mechanical strength and cell-matrix interactions. J Biomed Mater Res A 2007;80(2):362–71.
18. Balli E, Comelekoglu U, Yalin E, et al. Exposure to gamma rays induces early alterations in skin in rodents: mechanical, biochemical and structural responses. Ecotoxicol Environ Saf 2009;72(3):889–94.
19. Grimes M, Pembroke JT, McGloughlin T. The effect of choice of sterilisation method on the biocompatibility and biodegradability of SIS (small intestinal submucosa). Biomed Mater Eng 2005;15(1–2):65–71.

20. Noah EM, Chen J, Jiao X, et al. Impact of sterilization on the porous design and cell behavior in collagen sponges prepared for tissue engineering. Biomaterials 2002;23(14):2855–61.
21. Tyan YC, Liao JD, Lin SP, et al. The study of the sterilization effect of gamma ray irradiation of immobilized collagen polypropylene nonwoven fabric surfaces. J Biomed Mater Res A 2003;67(3):1033–43.
22. Barber FA, Herbert MA, Boothby MH. Ultimate tensile failure loads of a human dermal allograft rotator cuff augmentation. Arthroscopy 2008;24(1):20–4.
23. Barber FA, Herbert MA, Coons DA. Tendon augmentation grafts: biomechanical failure loads and failure patterns. Arthroscopy 2006;22(5):534–8.
24. Coons DA, Alan Barber F. Tendon graft substitutes-rotator cuff patches. Sports Med Arthrosc 2006;14(3):185–90.
25. Derwin KA, Baker AR, Spragg RK, et al. Commercial extracellular matrix scaffolds for rotator cuff tendon repair. Biomechanical, biochemical, and cellular properties. J Bone Joint Surg Am 2006;88(12):2665–72.
26. Aurora A, McCarron J, Iannotti JP, et al. Commercially available extracellular matrix materials for rotator cuff repairs: state of the art and future trends. J Shoulder Elbow Surg 2007;16(Suppl 5):S171–8.
27. Sakakeeny J. Defining the physicomechanical benefit of Tissuemend® in tendon augmentation surgeries. Department of Mechanical Engineering, Tufts University 2006; 71.
28. Macri L, Clark RA. Tissue engineering for cutaneous wounds: selecting the proper time and space for growth factors, cells and the extracellular matrix. Skin Pharmacol Physiol 2009;22(2):83–93.
29. Singer AJ, Clark RA. Cutaneous wound healing. N Engl J Med 1999;341(10):738–46.
30. Butler DL, Juncosa N, Dressler MR. Functional efficacy of tendon repair processes. Annu Rev Biomed Eng 2004;6:303–29.
31. Molloy T, Wang Y, Murrell G. The roles of growth factors in tendon and ligament healing. Sports Med 2003;33(5):381–94.
32. Macleod TM, Williams G, Sanders R, et al. Histological evaluation of Permacol as a subcutaneous implant over a 20-week period in the rat model. Br J Plast Surg 2005;58(4):518–32.
33. Petter-Puchner AH, Fortelny RH, Walder N, et al. Adverse effects associated with the use of porcine crosslinked collagen implants in an experimental model of incisional hernia repair. J Surg Res 2008;145(1):105–10.
34. Robinson TN, Clarke JH, Schoen J, et al. Major mesh-related complications following hernia repair: events reported to the Food and Drug Administration. Surg Endosc 2005;19(12):1556–60.
35. Rodriguez ER, Overman J. Preliminary results of a retrospective study utilizing a type 1 collagen xenograft in foot and ankle soft tissue reconstructive procedures. Long Beach (CA): American College of Foot and Ankle Surgeons; 2008.
36. Valentin JE, Badylak JS, McCabe GP, et al. Extracellular matrix bioscaffolds for orthopaedic applications. A comparative histologic study. J Bone Joint Surg Am 2006;88(12):2673–86.
37. Badylak S, Kokini K, Tullius B, et al. Strength over time of a resorbable bioscaffold for body wall repair in a dog model. J Surg Res 2001;99(2):282–7.
38. Nicholson GP, Breur GJ, Van Sickle D, et al. Evaluation of a crosslinked acellular porcine dermal patch for rotator cuff repair augmentation in an ovine model. J Shoulder Elbow Surg 2007;16(Suppl 5):S184–90.
39. Walton JR, Bowman NK, Khatib Y, et al. Restore orthobiologic implant: not recommended for augmentation of rotator cuff repairs. J Bone Joint Surg Am 2007;89(4):786–91.

40. Zheng MH, Chen J, Kirilak Y, et al. Porcine small intestine submucosa (SIS) is not an acellular collagenous matrix and contains porcine DNA: possible implications in human implantation. J Biomed Mater Res B Appl Biomater 2005;73(1):61–7.

41. Macher BA, Galili U. The Galalpha1,3Galbeta1,4GlcNAc-R (alpha-Gal) epitope: a carbohydrate of unique evolution and clinical relevance. Biochim Biophys Acta 2008;1780(2):75–88.

42. Galili U, Anaraki F, Thall A, et al. One percent of human circulating B lymphocytes are capable of producing the natural anti-Gal antibody. Blood 1993;82(8):2485–93.

43. Ansaloni L, Cambrini P, Catena F, et al. Immune response to small intestinal submucosa (surgisis) implant in humans: preliminary observations. J Invest Surg 2007;20(4):237–41.

44. Hwang K, Hwang JH, Park JH, et al. Experimental study of autologous cartilage, acellular cadaveric dermis, lyophilized bovine pericardium, and irradiated bovine tendon: applicability to nasal tip plasty. J Craniofac Surg 2007;18(3):551–8.

45. Gaertner WB, Bonsack ME, Delaney JP, et al. Experimental evaluation of four biologic prostheses for ventral hernia repair. J Gastrointest Surg 2007;11(10):1275–85.

46. Blatnik J, Jin J, Rosen M. Abdominal hernia repair with bridging acellular dermal matrix–an expensive hernia sac. Am J Surg 2008;196(1):47–50.

47. Jin J, Rosen MJ, Blatnik J, et al. Use of acellular dermal matrix for complicated ventral hernia repair: does technique affect outcomes? J Am Coll Surg 2007; 205(5):654–60.

48. Lee DK. Achilles tendon repair with acellular tissue graft augmentation in neglected ruptures. J Foot Ankle Surg 2007;46(6):451–5.

49. Lee DK. A preliminary study on the effects of acellular tissue graft augmentation in acute Achilles tendon ruptures. J Foot Ankle Surg 2008;47(1):8–12.

50. Liden BA, Simmons M. Histologic evaluation of a 6-month GraftJacket matrix biopsy used for Achilles tendon augmentation. J Am Podiatr Med Assoc 2009; 99(2):104–7.

51. Di Domenico LA, Williams K, Petrolla AF. Spontaneous rupture of the anterior tibial tendon in a diabetic patient: results of operative treatment. J Foot Ankle Surg 2008;47(5):463–7.

52. Berlet GC, Hyer CF, Lee TH, et al. Interpositional arthroplasty of the first MTP joint using a regenerative tissue matrix for the treatment of advanced hallux rigidus. Foot Ankle Int 2008;29(1):10–21.

53. Brigido SA. The use of an acellular dermal regenerative tissue matrix in the treatment of lower extremity wounds: a prospective 16-week pilot study. Int Wound J 2006;3(3):181–7.

54. Brigido SA, Boc SF, Lopez RC. Effective management of major lower extremity wounds using an acellular regenerative tissue matrix: a pilot study. Orthopedics 2004;27(Suppl 1):s145–9.

55. Mostow EN, Haraway GD, Dalsing M, et al. Effectiveness of an extracellular matrix graft (OASIS Wound Matrix) in the treatment of chronic leg ulcers: a randomized clinical trial. J Vasc Surg 2005;41(5):837–43.

56. Winters CL, Brigido SA, et al. A multicenter study involving the use of a human acellular dermal regenerative tissue matrix for the treatment of diabetic lower extremity wounds. Adv Skin Wound Care 2008;21(8):375–81.

57. Serena T. A novel fetal bovine matrix scaffold is rapidly incorporated into animal and human wounds resulting in wound bed stimulation. Wounds 2005;17(A42).

58. Kavros SJ. Treatment of chronic foot ulcerations in high risk individuals with primatrix. Fort Worth (TX): American Profession Wound Care Association (APWCA); 2008.

The Role of Collagen Bioscaffolds, Foamed Collagen, and Living Skin Equivalents in Wound Healing

Adam Landsman, DPM, PhD, FACFAS*, Drew Taft, DPM, Kevin Riemer, DPM

KEYWORDS

- Collagen • Soft tissue matrix • Wound • Diabetic foot ulcer
- Living skin equivalent

In its simplest form, the building blocks of skin can be distilled down to cellular and noncellular components. Cellular components include fibroblasts and keratinocytes, which are supported in a three-dimensional noncellular collagen matrix. Approximately 18 years ago, advanced biologics—consisting of various components of skin such as fibroblasts, keratinocytes, and decellularized collagen—became available for wound applications.

Collagen can be harvested from a variety of sources, including bovine and porcine skin, porcine intestine, equine pericardium, and other sources. Once harvested, each product is prepared in a proprietary process to remove the cellular components, leaving behind the native matrix. The removal of living and cellular components and cleansing varies from company to company, and has a direct influence on the degree of preservation of the native collagen structure. Although some manufacturers take great pains to preserve structure, others take a completely different approach, by either fractionating or foaming the collagen to retain the essence of a three-dimensional matrix, but not the overall native structure. Other companies use techniques to crosslink the collagen to add strength and durability. Still others laminate multiple layers to improve durability. There are potential advantages and disadvantages to each approach (see later discussion).

WOUND MANAGEMENT WITH COLLAGEN
Foamed Collagen

Foamed collagen is formed by breaking down collagen and combining it with cellulose. It aids in wound healing by providing substrate fragments to be incorporated

Division of Podiatric Surgery, Beth Israel Deaconess Medical Center, Baker 3, 1 Deaconess Road, Boston, MA 02215, USA
* Corresponding author.
E-mail address: alandsma@bidmc.harvard.edu (A. Landsman).

Clin Podiatr Med Surg 26 (2009) 525–533
doi:10.1016/j.cpm.2009.08.012
0891-8422/09/$ – see front matter © 2009 Elsevier Inc. All rights reserved.

into the wound bed and by absorbing matrix metalloproteases (MMPs) associated with chronic wounds and inflammation.[1,2] Normally, MMPs will degrade matrix collagen, further inhibiting the closure of the wound. Prisma and Promogran (Systagenix, North Yorkshire, UK) contain approximately 55% collagen and 44% cellulose (oxidized regenerated cellulose [ORC]), and, in the case of Prisma, 1% ionic silver bound to ORC. The addition of silver helps to reduce bacteria count. Biostep and Biostep Ag (Smith & Nephew, Largo, FL, USA) are similar products. They also contain collagen and carboxymethyl cellulose, and a sodium alginate that facilitates migration and tissue regeneration. Biostep also contains ethylenediaminetetraacetic acid (EDTA) which acts by inhibiting proteolytic enzymes in chronic wounds; thereby enhancing wound healing. There is also a silver-enhanced version to reduce bacteria count on the surface of the wound. Puracol Plus and Puracol Plus AG (Medline Industries, Mundeline, IL, USA) have taken a different approach to foamed collagen by providing a pure collagen product, without additives. They have retained the classic triple helix structure of the collagen, which aids in the binding of elastase, an upstream regulator of MMP action.[3–5]

Although there is variation in the specific mechanisms of action hypothesized by each specific brand, they have all proven themselves highly useful for the treatment of chronic wounds. Foamed collagens are effective for controlling exudates and reducing MMPs. They have been used in conjunction with negative pressure wound therapy (NPWT) to add collagen to the highly granular tissue that usually forms in association with this type of therapy. Wound healing requires a balance between collagen matrix assembly and cellular proliferation,[6] and foamed collagen can provide the matrix material to fill that need. **Fig. 1** demonstrates how this type of material can be used.

Fractionated and Powdered Collagen

Collagen processing involves the breakdown of natural bovine collagen into a form that is more easily handled. In addition, it has been hypothesized that fractionation allows the collagen to be incorporated more readily. Cellerate Rx (Wound Care Innovations, Ft. Lauderdale, FL, USA) is available as both a powder and compounded with a hydrogel. In these preparations, the collagen fibers are broken down to approximately 1/100 the length of unaltered fibers, resulting in elimination of essentially all crosslinking, thereby enhancing the rate of incorporation. However, the structural

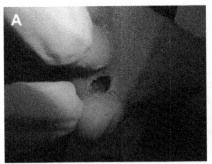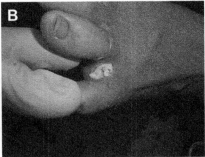

Fig.1. (A) Deep, tunneling wound in the fourth interspace on the foot of a patient with diabetes. The wound is debrided and presents with a clean, granular base. (B) The wound is packed with Biostep (Smith & Nephew, Largo, FL, USA) to fill the dead space, and stabilize the granulation tissue in the area.

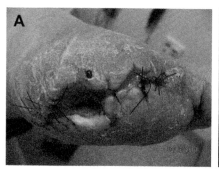
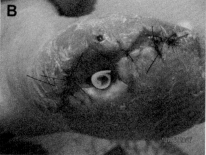

Fig. 2. (A) Another tunneling wound. Sheet collagen (Primatrix; TEI Biosciences Inc, Boston, MA) is rolled, and inserted into the wound. This material is dense and can provide a large amount of collagen to the wound surface. (B) The wound is filled with the collagen bioscaffold material.

benefits of collagen are lost. It is hypothesized that this material works as a bioactivator that uses collagen fragments to signal recruitment of macrophages and fibroblasts. Application is simple and can be repeated as needed.

Sheet Collagen and Compounded Collagen

Sheet collagen is known by many different names from soft tissue matrix to collagen bioscaffold. The primary difference between these materials is the relative percentage of collagen types, degree of crosslinking, tissue source, and form in which it is presented. See the article elsewhere in this issue regarding the technical differences between these materials.

Collagen bioscaffolds provide a matrix for stabilization of vascularized tissue and cellular components and play a role in chemotaxis to recruit fibroblasts and macrophages. These materials become incorporated into the wound bed at various rates, depending on a variety of factors, including the need for the collagen components provided, the degree of vascularity of the wound, and the presence of bacteria and MMPs. Although these materials are usually provided in a dry, sterile format, some

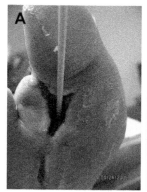
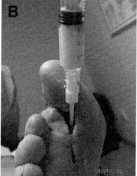
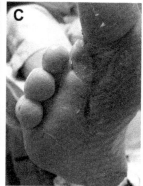

Fig. 3. (A) This wound extends several centimeters into the foot. (B) Flowable collagen (Integra Life Sciences Corp, Plainsboro, NJ, USA) is hydrated with saline using a specialized syringe with a large bore tip, and is deposited in the wound from deep to superficial, filling the area completely. (C) The wound is completely filled with the flowable collagen.

brands may be prehydrated. Dry materials will absorb exudates from the wounds. This may be beneficial in some instances. In other cases, the collagen can be fenestrated to implement drainage and aid in attachment of the collagen to the wound bed. **Fig. 2** shows the use of sheet collagen (Primatrix; TEI Biosciences Inc, Boston, MA, USA) on a chronic diabetic foot ulcer with a tunneling wound. In this case, the tunneling area of the wound is debrided, and the collagen material can be rolled and inserted into the tunnel. Within 2 weeks, following a single application, the tunneling area was completely filled. Alternatively, Graftjacket Xpress (Wright Medical Technologies, Memphis, TN, USA), a powdered human collagen, or Integra Flowable (Integra Life-sciences Corp, Plainsboro, NJ), a pulverized bovine collagen, can be compounded with sterile saline and mixed in a syringe. This viscous material can then be injected into the tunneling area (**Fig. 3**). It helps to close the tunneling wound by displacing pooled fluid, while stimulating chemotaxis to attract fibroblasts and macrophages to the area.

Although sheet collagen bioscaffolds can be simply laid across or stitched into the surface of a wound, it can also be used in conjunction with NPWT. In this application,

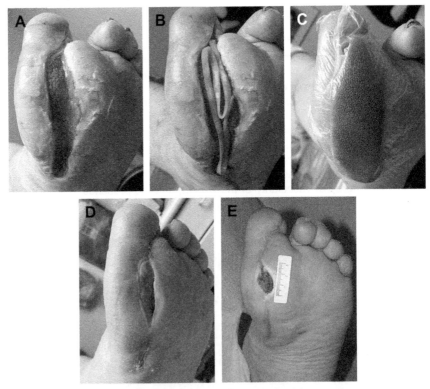

Fig. 4. (*A*) A large (>80 cm^2) wound previously treated with negative pressure wound therapy is ready to receive collagen. (*B*) Primatrix Fetal bovine collagen (TEI Biosciences Inc, Boston, MA, USA) is available in strips and is laid across the wound surface. (*C*) A non-adherent, highly fenestrated material is applied over the collagen and the sponge used in the application of negative pressure wound therapy is laid directly over that. (*D*) After several weeks, progression of the wound is apparent. (*E*) Following three applications of collagen, the wound continues to improve.

the deeper wound is first layered with collagen, then with a highly fenestrated nonadherent material. On top of this, the NPWT interface (sponge, in this case) is laid on top. As a result, the collagen becomes rapidly integrated into the wound bed as the vascular tissue rapidly penetrates it. An example of this technique is shown in **Fig. 4**, demonstrating rapid closure of a wound measuring approximately 80 cm^2, initially, which achieved total closure in approximately 12 weeks following three applications of collagen strips.

Composite Collagen Bioscaffolds

A unique type of collagen bioscaffold is the bilayer wound dressing. Integra Bilayer Matrix Wound Dressing (Integra Lifesciences Corp, Plainsboro, NJ, USA) consists of a pulverized bovine collagen soft tissue matrix bonded to a silicone sheet. The multi-layered structure is easy to handle and can be stitched over the wound site (**Fig. 5**). The silicone material is left in place while the collagen material is gradually dissolved or incorporated into the wound bed. It has been suggested that the silicone portion of the dressing retains moisture in the wound bed. Moisture preservation is a critical element in wound healing, which allows transport of enzymes and cells, and prevents dessication.[7]

Implanted Collagen as an Adjunct to Wound Healing

Recently, collagen bioscaffolds have been used for fat pad augmentation with great success. In particular, non-crosslinked and minimally crosslinked collagen bioscaffolds have been shown to cause minimal inflammatory reactions and appear to be well integrated into the deep tissues. Deep implantation of collagen and collagen pieces can be used to build up tissues adjacent to bony prominences, to help reduce the focal pressures associated with diabetic foot ulcers or decubitus heel ulcers. **Fig. 6** shows a patient with a midfoot ulcer secondary to Charcot neuroarthropathy with the tissue adjacent to the prominence built up to take pressure off the area. **Fig. 7** shows a heel decubitus ulcer that was treated with resection of the necrotic tissue and a partial calcanectomy. Before wound closure, fetal bovine collagen was implanted

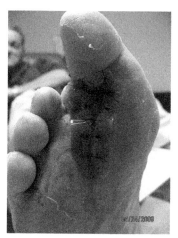

Fig. 5. The wound is covered with Integra Bilayer Wound dressing (Integra Life Sciences Corp, Plainsboro, NJ, USA). This material will remain in place until healed or the silicone portion separates.

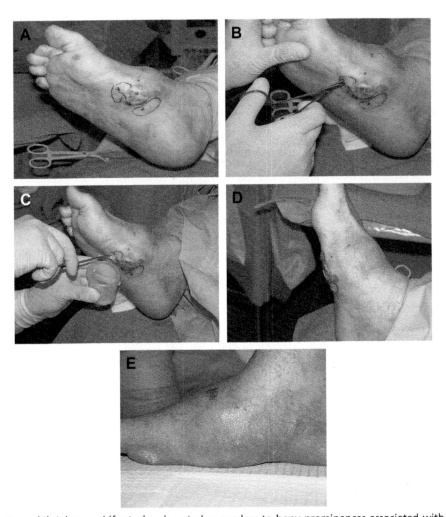

Fig. 6. (*A*) A large midfoot ulcer is noted, secondary to bony prominences associated with Charcot. Purple areas mark depressed areas adjacent to the ulcer site. (*Courtesy of Dr. J. Karr, Lakeland, FL*). (*B*) Using a hemostat, the depressed areas are opened through a stab incision to create a space for insertion of collagen. (*C*) Fetal bovine collagen (Primatrix; TEI, Boston, MA, USA) is chopped into small pieces and inserted through the tiny openings to pack and elevate the periwound areas. (*D*) Once packed, the prominence has been eliminated, leaving a cushioned, flat surface. (*E*) With weight bearing, the fill adjacent to the ulcer site can be appreciated.

to cover the bone and prevent adhesions. In the final picture, the soft tissues have a full, well-padded appearance.

Living Skin Equivalents and Living Human Cadaveric Skin

Living skin equivalents are living tissues grown in the laboratory and contain some of the components of human skin. Currently, there are two living skin equivalents available in the United States that are approved by the Food and Drug Administration for treatment of diabetic foot ulcers. Apligraf (Organogenesis, Canton, MA, USA) and DermaGraft (Advanced BioHealing, La Jolla, CA, USA) are created in the laboratory from

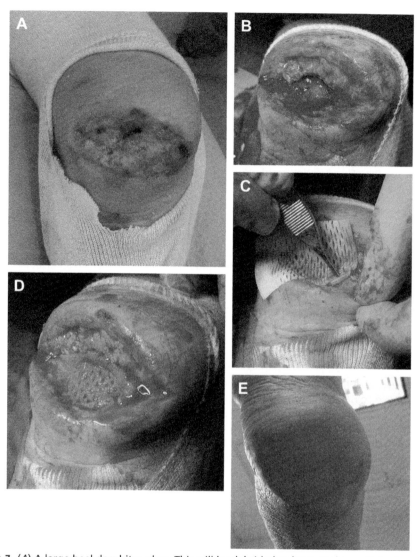

Fig. 7. (A) A large heel decubitus ulcer. This will be debrided to bone and a partial calcanectomy will be performed. (B) The wound has been excised and the surface of the calcaneous has been exposed and debrided. (C) SurgiMend bovine collagen (TEI Biosciences Inc, Boston, MA, USA) is fenestrated and applied over the surface of the bone to prevent adhesions between the bone and overlying skin, and to enhance healing through chemotaxis. (D) Collagen graft is stitched in place and is ready for wound closure. (E) Resolution of the ulcer site is complete 5 weeks after surgery.

living human tissues. DermaGraft contains fibroblasts attached to an absorbable substrate. It is applied to the surface of diabetic foot ulcers to deliver growth factors. It arrives as a frozen product and requires a specific defrosting process before application. Apligraf consists of fibroblasts and keratinocytes attached to a bovine collagen scaffold. It also delivers growth factors to the surface of the wound, along with a collagen substrate. Both materials have been shown to aid in the closure of ulcers.

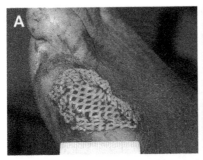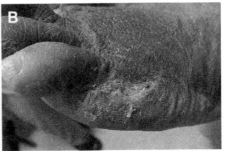

Fig. 8. (A) TheraSkin (LifeNet Health, Virginia Beach, VA, USA) living human cadaveric split thickness skin graft is stitched into position over the wound. (B) Two weeks later, the wound is completely healed.

More recently, living human cadaveric skin, harvested within 12 hours of death by a tissue bank and cryopreserved, has reemerged as a strong alternative to the laboratory-created skin equivalents. Sold under the name, TheraSkin (LifeNet Health, Virginia Beach, VA, USA), these products have been proven to be safe and contain the full array of components found in native skin—because it is living human skin. They are durable and will release growth factors and collagen components to the wound bed to stimulate healing. Living cadaveric skin is handled and applied in the same way as any split thickness skin graft. It can be stitched over the wound and left in place until closure is achieved (**Fig. 8**).

Whenever the subject of living skin equivalents and living cadaveric skin is raised, questions about rejection and stimulation of immune responses is not far behind. In fact, these materials ultimately are attacked by our bodies, leading to lysis of living cells and release of growth factors. The immune response triggered by implantation of these materials is short-lived because the graft has no support structure of its own and dies as its inert components become incorporated.[8,9]

In order to preserve the living tissues of the implant as long as possible, it is essential that the clinician select a dressing material that helps to preserve and sustain the implant. In addition, nonadherent dressing materials may help avoid unintentional disruption of the implant. Some manufacturers (ie, Advanced BioHealing, manufacturers of DermaGraft) also recommend avoiding petroleum-based dressing to diminish the risk of maceration. Wounds that are desiccated or macerated heal more slowly and are more susceptible to complications. In order to meet these broad demands, dressings such as TheraGauze (Soluble Systems, Inc, Newport News, VA, USA), an advanced polymer dressing that is nonadherent and capable of either donating or absorbing moisture from the wound bed, has been shown to work well.[10] With TheraGauze, wounds achieve proper moisture balance, heal more quickly, and heal more frequently. Preliminary data indicates that the use of this moisture regulating dressing will reduce the number of living skin equivalents necessary to achieve wound closure in patients with diabetic foot ulcers.[10]

SUMMARY

Healing of complex wounds is a continually evolving science. Issues of excess mechanical forces, bacteria load, inflammation, diminished growth factors, and, of course, a lack of collagen will influence outcomes. Collagen serves as an important tool because it provides an essential building block necessary for complete wound healing. In this article, it is demonstrated that collagen implants may also serve to control mechanical loads. Dispersing mechanical forces around areas of bony prominences is something that has been tried with many materials in the past, from injectable silicone to hyaluronic acid. The advantage of using collagen in this application appears to be the ability to integrate the material into native tissues for a longer lasting and more durable repair.

Based upon the authors' experiences, it is clear that there are certain areas where the addition of collagen is particularly beneficial. Most notable is where the wound is highly granular and vascular. When collagen is applied here, it will stabilize the vascular tissue and help to develop the sturdy matrix necessary to support continued wound closure.

Many different types of collagen products are now available to the physicians involved in wound care. This article did not discuss the area of porcine intestinal mucosa or equine pericardium. Although these materials are widely used in wound care, they are typically more heavily cross-linked and, as such, are more resistant to enzymatic degradation and incorporation into native tissues. In addition, collagen implants are typically viewed as advanced wound dressings. Specifically, it is perceived that their primary benefit is to regulate the biochemical environment of the wound. In theory, this is similar to the way that a thin layer of native skin would act. However, collagen does many things that an advanced wound dressing cannot—particularly as it relates to stimulation of chemotaxis, mitosis, and angiogenesis.

REFERENCES

1. Wysocki AB, Staniano-Coico L, Grinnell F. Wound fluid from chronic leg ulcers contains elevated levels of metalloproteinases MMP-2 and MMP-9. J Invest Dermatol 1993;101:64–8.
2. Hart J. Inflammation 2: its role in the healing of chronic wounds. J Wound Care 2002;11:245–9.
3. Edwards JV, Howley P, Cohen IK, et al. In vitro inhibition of human neutrophil elastase by oleic acid albumin formulations from derivatized cotton wound dressings. Int J Pharm 2004;284:1–12.
4. Chen SM, Ward SI, Olutoye OO, et al. Ability of chronic wound fluids to degrade peptide growth factors is associated with increased levels of elastase activity and diminished levels of proteinase inhibitors. Wound Repair Regen 1997;5:23–32.
5. Zhu YK, Liu XD, Skold CM, et al. Synergistic neutrophil elastase-cytokine interaction degrades collagen in three-dimensional culture. Am J Physiol Lung Cell Mol Physiol 2001;281:L868–78.
6. Landsman A, Roukis TS, DeFronzo DJ, et al. Living cells or collagen matrix: which is more beneficial in the treatment of diabetic foot ulcers? Wounds 2008;20(5): 111–6.
7. Eaglstein WH. Moist wound healing with occlusive dressings: a clinical focus. Dermatol Surg 2001;27:175–81.
8. Bravo D, Rigley TH, Gibran N, et al. Effect of storage and preservation methods on viability in transplantable human skin allografts. Burns 2000;26:367–78.
9. Spence RJ, Wong L. The enhancement of wound healing with human skin allograft. Surg Clin North Am 1997;77(3):731–45.
10. Landsman A. "Optimizing adherence of skin grafts, living skin equivalents, and collagen bioscaffolds with a moisture regulating wound dressing." Oral Abstract presented at the 2009 annual Scientific Meeting of the American Podiatric Medical Association. Toronto: Canada; July 30, 2009.

Bioscaffolds and the Reconstruction of Ligaments and Tendons in the Foot and Ankle

Jeremy J. Cook, DPM, MPH*, Emily A. Cook, DPM, MPH

KEYWORDS

• Bioscaffold • Matrix • Collagen • Foot • Ligament

A variety of podiatric surgical pathologie involve or rely on the integrity of a tendon or ligament for successful treatment. This holds true for forefoot procedures such as the Jones tenosuspension, and more complex reconstructive procedures such as lateral ankle joint stabilizations discussed elsewhere in this issue. When native tissues are inadequate and require augmentation, alternative options become necessary. Recently, connective tissue engineering has led to significant advances in this field and may offer advantages over traditional options. Several technologies fall under the heading of connective tissue engineering. The scope of this article is limited to the subgroup of connective tissue alternatives known as bioscaffolds. These products are compared with one another and to traditional alternatives. Specific preimplantation conditioning steps to optimize outcomes are presented. An overview of these materials in clinical research, as they relate to musculoskeletal surgery in the foot and ankle is presented.

INDICATIONS

Tendon healing is comprised of four stages that span a period beginning just hours after an injury, ending weeks to months later.[1,2] The overall healing process closely mimics wound healing. Initially, an inflammatory reaction occurs within 72 hours of the insult and lasts up to 7 days. Infiltration of cells from the endotenon, epitenon, and peritenon form a stabilizing fibroblastic callus while the local inflammatory cascade is active. The next phase lasts 7 to 14 days and is marked by proliferation of endotenon cells and increased production of disorganized collagen fibers. During this time, the tendon is still quite weak and requires protection in the form of a cast or splint. The third stage includes further collagen production but in a more organized

Division of Podiatric Surgery, Department of Surgery, Harvard Medical School, Beth Israel Deaconess Medical Center, One Deaconess Road, Boston, MA 02215, USA
* Corresponding author.
E-mail address: jcook2@bidmc.harvard.edu (J.J. Cook).

Clin Podiatr Med Surg 26 (2009) 535–543
doi:10.1016/j.cpm.2009.07.004
0891-8422/09/$ – see front matter © 2009 Elsevier Inc. All rights reserved.

podiatric.theclinics.com

manner. Passive range of motion may be initiated at this stage that enhances the alignment of fibers along the long axis of the tendon. Finally, the maturation phase will begin after approximately 5 weeks postinjury. At this point, collagen production is greatly reduced and remodeling of the site becomes the primary activity.[1,2]

Hui and colleagues[3] reported that tendon remodeling is often incomplete and poorly mimics the original structure. The new structure has significantly increased cellular density compared to native uninjured tissues, which negatively impacts the tensile strength of the tendon.[4,5] It is believed that the tensile strength may be reduced by as much as one-third for months after an injury.[4] The inferior mechanical quality of the tissue is believed to be directly related to the relative inactivity of native cells and modest vascular supply.[6,7] Furthermore, when tendons and ligaments are subjected to prolonged inflammation, they suffer degenerative changes that can reduce the success of primary repair and compromise fixation.[8] When the ability of the native tissue to support fixation is compromised, engineered tissue augmentation is most appropriate.[9] Several studies[10–12] have suggested that key features desired in a tendon or ligament implant should include blood vessels and collagen fibers and promote cellular migration and native tissue ingress. Ideally, this should occur in the absence of a significant inflammatory response.

Additional bioscaffold augmentation indications are poorly described in the literature. This lack of definitive indications is mainly because of the novelty of the technology and the paucity of clinical research. One contributing factor may be the fact that bioscaffolds are considered to be a medical device and, therefore, are not subject to the same level of scrutiny as pharmaceutical therapies. Because of this, indications for their use are based on level 4 and 5 data in most instances and in all research related to the foot and ankle.[13] When there is inadequate tendon or ligament length, strength, or girth, tissue augmentation with bioscaffold is an option that can be considered. A thorough preoperative examination, which may include MRI or tenograms, can permit a greater degree of detail for planning purposes. However, inadequate tendon or ligament length or girth may only become evident intraoperatively. In some cases, the native tissue itself appears weak and atrophied with poor ability to retain sutures. This is particularly common in patients with a traumatic or chronic disease state. Augmentation offers a solid anchoring point, which potentially provides load sharing that can protect the repair site.

TISSUE AUGMENTATION OPTIONS

Depending on the procedure, choices are available for augmentation of tendons or ligaments. Autograft augmentation has the major advantage of being fresh and histologically compatible. However, autograft harvesting involves additional morbidity from the donor site, may result in new problematic deformities, or—as in the setting of Ehlers-Danlos syndrome—the tissue may be otherwise compromised. Mechanical testing on commonly used autografts for lateral ankle stabilization procedures has been performed, the characteristics of which can be seen in **Table 1**.[14]

Synthetic materials have been widely available since the late 1980s and are typically made from polymers. Although very strong and durable, their primary limitation has been related to biocompatibility.[13] Long-term results following use of these materials have shown complications ranging from severe foreign body reactions to complete implant failure.[13] The largest clinical trial involving a synthetic scaffold in podiatric surgery is the Leed-Keio implant.[15] This was designed to simulate an anterior cruciate ligament with mechanical testing that demonstrated a strength of 780 ± 200 Newtons

Table 1
Biomechanical characteristics of native tissues in the ankle stabilization

Native Tissue	Cross-Sectional Area (mm²)	Load to Failure (N)	Ultimate Strain (%)	Ankle Stabilization Procedure
Peroneus longus	2240 ± 530	1342 ± 135	34.3–63.7	Hambley[36]
Split Achilles tendon	3810 ± 3460	1013 ± 278	33.7–90.3	Storen[37]
Fascia	2240 ± 830	596 ± 265	36.3–95.4	Elmslie[38]
Corium	4550 ± 1420	496 ± 122	46.9–46.9	Gschwend[39]
Plantaris	210 ± 80	93.8 ± 14.9	21.2–34.8	Weber[40]
ATF	2620 ± 600, NA	150, 139	197.5–252.5, NA	Brostrom[41]
PTF	NA	261	NA	—
CF	NA	346	NA	—

Abbreviations: ATF, anterior talofibular ligament; CF, alcaneal fibular ligament; N, newtons; NA, not applicable; PTF, posterior talofibular ligament.

Data from Bohnsack M, Surie B, Wulker N. Biomechanical properties of commonly used autogenous transplants in the surgical treatment of chronic lateral ankle instability. Foot Ankle Int 2002;23(7):661–4.[14]

Data from Attarian DE, McCrackin HJ, DeVito DP, et al. Biomechanical characteristics of human ankle ligaments. Foot Ankle 1985;6:54–8.

(N).[13] In this retrospective cohort study, lateral collateral ligaments were augmented and found to have few complications.

Tendon allograft provides biomaterial qualities that closely mimic the recipient's tissue, but is costly. It is also believed that the age of the donor has an impact on tensile strength. Allografts in patients over 64 years old were compared with a group under 50 years old and found that ultimate tensile strength was 17% lower in the older group.[16] Another alternative and the focus of the remainder of this article are a subgroup of engineered tissues called bioscaffolds. They are also commonly referred to as extracellular matrices or acellular collagen tissue. Bioscaffolds are essentially a collagen matrix derived from either human or animal sources. The type of source tissue can be further categorized as dermal, submucosal, or pericardial. The cellular elements of each of these tissues are removed by proprietary methods leaving a mixture of elastin, proteoglycans, and collagen. Although the content and ratio of collagen types varies between bioscaffolds, type I is the most abundant.[17] Furthermore, the manufacturers of bioscaffolds report that the surfaces of these products are biologically active.[13]

BIOSCAFFOLDS

A variety of bioscaffold options is available with several products taking advantage of the similarities between wound and tendon healing. As of early January 2009, there are eight Food and Drug Administration-approved bioscaffolds. The major properties of commonly used bioscaffolds can be seen in **Table 2**. Bioscaffolds serve two primary functions in tendon and ligament augmentation. The first is their enhancement of healing in the pathologic setting. This is believed to occur by stimulating angiogenesis and promoting host cellular migration and proliferation.[18] Snyder and colleagues[19] retrieved a biopsy from a tendon augmented with a bioscaffold 3 months after implantation in a 62-year-old man with a chronic rotator cuff tear. Histologic examination of the biopsy demonstrated significant incorporation of native cells and blood vessels with scant inflammatory reaction. Collagen from the bioscaffold was arranged parallel

Table 2
General and biomechanical features of available bioscaffolds

Name	Tissue Source	Thickness (mm)	Cross-linkage or Lamination	Load to Failure (N)[17]	Elongation at Failure (mm)[23]	Strain (%)[23]	Incorporation[21,42]
GraftJacket	Human dermis	2.0 1.4 1.0	None	229 ± 72 182 ± 50.2 157 ± 37.8	16–28	53%–93%	PI16
Tissuemend	Fetal bovine dermis	1.1 1.2	None	76 ± 21.5 70 ± 13.3	11–16 —	37%–53%	PI16
Bioblanket	Adult bovine dermis	1.0	Cross-linked	NA	NA	NA	NA
Zimmer or Permacol	Porcine dermis	1.0	Cross-linked	128 ± 26.3	NA	NA	UI16
Restore	Porcine SIS	1.0	10 Layers	38.2 ± 2.8	6.6–7.5	22%–25%	CI8
Cuffpatch	Porcine SIS	1.0 0.30[22]	Cross-linked 8 Layers	32 ± 4.1 26 ± 12.1[22]	— 6.0–6.6[22]	20%–22%	NCI8
Encuff patch	Bovine or porcine pericardium	1.0	Cross-linked	NA	NA	NA	NA
OrthoADAPT[22]	Equine pericardium	0.74 0.68 0.75	FX: Fully PX: Partial MX: Minimal	25.5 ± 18.2 12.9 ± 7.3 27.4 ± 4.2	— 5.7 ± 2.1 —	— 8–17.2% —	NA

Abbreviations: CI8, completely incorporated 8-weeks postimplantation; FX, fully cross-linked; MX, minimally cross-linked; NA, not applicable; NCI8, Near completely incorporated 8-weeks postimplantation; PX, partially cross-linked; P16, partially incorporated at 16-weeks postimplantation; SIS, small intestinal submucosa; UI16, unincorporated at 16-weeks postimplantation.

with native tendon fibers. Additionally, the incorporated tissue more closely resembled new tissue as opposed to scar formation, which suggests regeneration rather than repair. Similar findings have been found in a biopsy of a reinforced Achilles tendon 6 months postimplantation.[20] Histologic evaluation demonstrated near complete incorporation of the bioscaffold with widespread infiltration by native tissues and little evidence of inflammation.

There is variation in the induction properties in each of the bioscaffolds.[21] Graft-Jacket (Wright Medical Technology, Arlington, TN, USA) induces primarily collagen formation, while Tissuemend (TEI Biosciences, Boston, MA, USA) also demonstrated induction of adipocytes. Similarly, Restore (DePuy Orthopedics, Warsaw, IN, USA) had collagen and adipocyte formation, but to a lesser degree, and also induced muscle cell formation.

Successful incorporation and minimal immunologic response may not always be evident and can vary between each of the bioscaffolds.[21] Few studies have been conducted which evaluate the differences between bioscaffolds regarding immunologic response and incorporation. One such study was performed by Valentin and colleagues.[21] They used a musculotendinous rat model that compared five of the most commonly marketed bioscaffolds to an autologous tissue graft. Within each group, the rats were divided into different harvest and evaluation intervals. This ranged from 2 days postimplantation to 112 days postimplantation and included seven sample periods for each graft group. Evaluation consisted of semiquantitative histologic analysis in four areas: (1) cellular infiltration, (2) multinucleated giant cells, (3) vascularity, and (4) connective tissue organization. Their findings showed that human dermis and porcine submucosal bioscaffolds had the greatest amount of cellular infiltration.

Multinucleated giant cells, a marker of foreign body reaction, were noted in the human and porcine dermis samples while only one of the porcine submucosal scaffolds initiated this response. The other porcine submucosal scaffold along with the bovine dermis and autologous graft never manifested this response. Vascular ingress was greatest in the autologous graft and both porcine submucosal scaffolds. At the 16-week interval, only the porcine dermis bioscaffold showed an absence of new host extracellular matrix formation.

The second function that bioscaffolds serve is as a structural support for the healing tissue and as an additional point of fixation.[8] Mechanical properties of bioscaffolds are important as they are intended to augment a weak portion of the reconstructed tendon or ligament. The variations in graft source and processing can have significant influence on the strength of the product. Barber and colleagues[17] performed load to failure testing on a variety of bioscaffolds. Eight bioscaffolds, manufactured by five different companies were evaluated. GraftJacket and Tissuemend were represented by variations in thickness (example is 1.1 mm and 1.2 mm thickness forms of Tissuement) were separately tested. Although the samples were not pretensioned, each bioscaffold was hydrated per manufacturer guidelines. The results showed mean load to failure rang from 32 N to 229 N. When limiting this to only 1.0 mm thickness forms, the range narrowed to 32 N to 157 N. Guiot and colleagues[22] similarly conducted mechanical tests of CuffPatch (Arthrotek, Warsaw, IN, USA), and OrthoADAPT (Pegasus Biologic, Irvine, CA, USA)with varying degrees of cross-linkage. In this study, the thickness was less than 1.0 mm but represented the standard product characteristics of OrthoADAPT. It was noted that mean load to failure ranged from 13 N to 27 N with the partially cross-linked having the lowest average and the minimally cross-linked providing the upper bound. This seems counterintuitive because one of the primary justifications of cross-linkage is that it provides greater strength.[22] The

CuffPatch load to failure was only slightly less in the 0.3 mm thickness versus the 1.0 mm thickness seen in Barber's study. Finally, Derwin and colleagues[23] noted that the load-sharing contribution of bioscaffolds is likely far less significant than the supportive healing properties.[23]

Preparation and Insertion of the Bioscaffolds

Preimplantation handling of the bioscaffold is important and largely depends on the scope and intended use of the tissue. One element of preparation that is nearly universal relates to pre-tensioning of the bioscaffold. Much like autographs, bioscaffolds have a viscoelastic nature that mandates prestressing before they can be implanted; otherwise gradual postimplantation lengthening can occur which compromises patient outcome.[24] Derwin and colleagues[23] found that bioscaffolds required a 10% to 30% stretch before they began to carry any significant load. Several methods exist for accomplishing this and can be as simple as applying maximum manual force to using a commercial tensiometer. Lee and colleagues[24] performed a study using cadaveric porcine models that compared various tensioning methods. After pretensioning, the tendons were subjected to cyclic load to failure. They were also able to determine the additional lengthening that occurred in each tendon after the cyclic loading. Manually pretensioned tendons had a mean displacement of 15.6%, while those subjected to the tensiometer had a mean displacement of 10.9%. Tendons prepared with the tensiometer also had a mean load to failure 8.8% higher than the manually tensioned group ($P<.001$). The differences are attributed to be likely due to the difference in duration and force applied to the two groups. Within the manually tensioned group, force ranged between 45 to 65 N for 30 to 50 seconds. While tendons prepared with the tensiometer were subjected to 89 N of force for 15 minutes. Landsman[25] reported that that bioscaffolds that were prestressed between 30% to 40% resulted in as much as a doubling of the load to failure. Despite these findings, the amount of force applied and duration is not well defined. In the Lee study, the investigators found that 87.7% of graft elongation occurred during the first 5 minutes of tensioning relative to the same specimen after 30 minutes of equal force. The benefits of pretensioning are also time dependent.[26] Following periods of unloading, the tendon can begin to contract and therefore lose the benefits of pretensioning. A study by O'Brien suggested that this begins to occur after being in an unloaded state for 15 minutes. Graf and colleagues[27] found that the properties of pretensioning were maintained for as long as 30 minutes after preparation. In summary, pretensioning is an important aspect of tendon augmentation. Although duration and force specifics are still under review, pretensioning should be performed in these cases with all efforts made by the surgeon to minimize the unloading time before implantation.

Intraoperative storage of bioscaffold tendon grafts is another element that should be considered. Some surgeons will soak the graft in normal saline to prevent desiccation and improve pliability of the material. This is considered acceptable practice in most situations. However, is not recommended if the graft is intended to be passed through an osseous tunnel. Rogell and colleagues[28] examined the influence of submerging cadaveric human tendons in a basin of normal saline versus wrapping the grafts in saline-soaked gauze. They found that tendons submerged in the basin had enlarged and required 11.7% more force to pass through an osseous tunnel as compared with the samples wrapped in moist gauze. They noted that this was also time dependent as tendons submerged for 20 minutes had a 17.1% increase in pull through force compared with the shortest period. They concluded that the risk of damage to the graft, such as delamination, was reduced by facilitating low-resistance graft passage.

Bioscaffolds in Foot and Ankle

Few clinical trials have been published in peer-reviewed literature with regard to outcomes of bioscaffold tissues in foot and ankle surgery. Applications have been published on use for wound care; however, that topic is beyond the scope of this article. As of January 2009, only six articles have discussed use of one of these scaffolds in a clinical study. Two of the six articles are case reports; the remainder are retrospective cohorts.[20,29–33] All six articles discussed use of the GraftJacket or Pegasus products, and most involved surgical care of acute and chronic injuries of the Achilles tendon. In total, they included 93 cases with follow-up ranging from 6 to 42 months. No recurrence or implant-related complications were noted in any of the study subjects.

Cadaveric mechanical testing of the human Achilles tendon found that the mean load to failure among specimens was approximately 5100 N.[34] The load to failure forces are not the expected value of typical activity following surgery. It is fairer to anticipate that 50% of native tissue value would be expected. The load to failure seen in these artificial tissues ranges between 12.9 ± 7.3 N (OrthoADAPT PX) and 229 ± 72 N (GraftJacket). None of these specimens had been prestressed during load to failure testing. Given the proposed benefit of prestressing by Landsman, the load to failure could be as much as 458 N, representing 9% of the observed load to failure of the Achilles tendon. This would greatly exceed the mechanical strength of native lateral ankle ligaments. This supports the concept that these tissues are intended as a bridge until complete healing occurs; not as a permanent replacement.

A number of potential applications for bioscaffolds have been reported. Rubin and Schweitzer[35] presented several applications ranging from posterior tibial tendon repair to augmentation of the extensor hallucis longus. They also presented several technique suggestions in using these tissues. Though extensive in its presentation, follow-up of these applications were not detailed and further information in terms of efficacy cannot be provided.

A study by Lee[33] used GraftJacket and OrthoADAPT in 50 patients with stage II posterior tibial tendon dysfunction. The author augmented the posterior tibial tendon with one of the bioscaffolds. Unfortunately, direct comparative analysis was not included, and neither was a control. Mean follow up was 24.6 months with a range of 10 to 42 months. MRI images taken at least 24-months postoperatively demonstrated no evidence of residual inflammation. The complication rate for this study was 16% and consisted of eight superficial wound infections successfully treated with oral antibiotics. Application consisted of intratendinous weaving or wrap-around of the augmented structure.

SUMMARY

Several commercially available alternatives are already in the marketplace. The advantages and disadvantages of these products have been discussed with emphasis on appropriate preparation of the implant. Few prospective trials have been conducted in tendon and ligament repair. This is particularly true in the case of foot and ankle surgery. Bioscaffolds offer improved incorporation and compatibility over synthetics. They are typically inferior to synthetics with regard to mechanical strength, although this deficiency can be minimized by proper preparation before implantation. These grafts are too weak to be used in isolation, but offer an increase in mechanical strength, which is modest within tendons but far more comparable to ligaments. Further clinical trials are warranted to determine optimal patient selection and whether differences between implants offer significant advantages.

REFERENCES

1. Platt MA. Tendon repair and healing. Clin Podiatr Med Surg 2005;22:553–60.
2. Armagan O, Shereff M. Tendon injury and repair. In: Myerson M, editor, Foot and ankle disorders, vol. 2. Philadelphia: WB Saunders; 2000. p. 942–71.
3. Hui JHP, Ouyang HW, Hutmacher DW, et al. Mesenchymal stem cells in musculoskeletal tissue engineering: a review of recent advances in national university of Singapore. Ann Acad Med Singap 2005;34:206–12.
4. Leadbetter WB. Cell matrix response in tendon injury. Clin Sports Med 1992;2(3):533–77.
5. Liu SH, Yang RS, Al-Shaikh R, et al. Collagen in tendon, ligament, and bone healing. Clin Orthop Relat Res 1995;318:265–78.
6. Schulze-Tanzil G, Mobasheri A, Clegg PD, et al. Cultivation of human tenocytes in high-density culture. Histochem Cell Biol 2004;122:219–28.
7. Heinemeier K, Langberg H, Olesen JL, et al. Role of TGF-b1 in relation to exercise-induced type I collagen synthesis in human tendinous tissue. J Appl Physiol 2003;95:2390–7.
8. Fini M, Torricelli P, Giavaresi G, et al. In vitro study comparing two collageneous membranes in view of their clinical application for rotator cuff tendon regeneration. J Orthop Res 2007;25(1):98–107.
9. Calve S, Dennis RG, Kosnik PE, et al. Engineering of functional tendon. Tissue Eng 2004;10:755–61.
10. Arnoczky SP, Warren RF, Minei JP. Replacement of the anterior cruciate ligament using a synthetic prosthesis. An evaluation of graft biology in the dog. Am J Sports Med 1986;14:1–6.
11. Hoffmann MW, Wening JV, Apel R, et al. Repair and reconstruction of the anterior cruciate ligament by the "sandwich technique." A comparative microangiographic and histological study in the rabbit. Arch Orthop Trauma Surg 1993;112:113–20.
12. Jackson DW, Grood ES, Arnoczky SP, et al. Cruciate reconstruction using freeze dried anterior cruciate ligmant allograft and a ligament augmentation device (LAD). An experiemental study in a goat model. Am J Sports Med 1987;15(6):528–38.
13. Chen J, Xu J, Wang A, et al. Scaffolds for tendon and ligament repair: review of the efficacy of commercial products. Expert Rev Med Devices 2009;6:61–73.
14. Bohnsack M, Surie B, Wulker N. Biomechanical properties of commonly used autogenous transplants in the surgical treatment of chronic lateral ankle instability. Foot Ankle Int 2002;23(7):661–4.
15. Usami N, Inokuchi S, Hiraishi E, et al. Clinical applications of artificial ligaments for ankle instability—long-term follow up. J Long Term Eff Med Implants 2000;10(4):239–50.
16. Johnson GA, Tramaglini DM, Levine RE, et al. Tensile and viscoelastic properties of human patellar tendon. J Orthop Res 1994;12(6):796–803.
17. Barber FA, Herbert MA, Coons DA. Tendon augmentation grafts: biomechanical failure loads and failure patterns. Arthroscopy 2006;22(5):534–8.
18. Hing KA. Bone repair in the twenty-first century: biology, chemistry or engineering? Philos Trans R Soc Lond A 2004;362:2821–50.
19. Snyder SJ, Arnoczky SP, Bond JL, et al. Histologic evaluation of a biopsy specimen obtained 3 months after rotator cuff augmentation with GraftJacket matrix. Arthroscopy 2009;25(3):329–33.
20. Liden BA, Simmons M. Histologic evaluation of a 6-month GraftJacket matrix biopsy used for Achilles tendon augmentation. J Am Podiatr Med Assoc 2009;99(2):104–7.

21. Valentin JE, Badylak JS, McCabe GP, et al. Extracellular matrix bioscaffolds for orthopedic applications. J Bone Joint Surg Am 2006;88(12):2673–86.
22. Johnson W, Inamasu J, Yantzer B, et al. Comparative in vitro biomechanical evaluation of two soft tissue defect products. J Biomed Mater Res B Appl Biomater 2007 [Epub ahead of print].
23. Derwin KA, Baker AR, Spragg RK, et al. Commercial extracellular matrix scaffolds for rotator cuff tendon repair. Biomechanical, biochemical, and cellular properties. J Bone Joint Surg Am 2006;88(12):2665–72.
24. Lee CH, Huang GS, Chao KH, et al. Differential pretensions of a flexor tendon graft for anterior cruciate ligament reconstruction: a biomechanical comparison in a porcine knee model. Arthroscopy 2005;21(5):540–6.
25. Landsman A. Mechanical loading of collagen bioscaffolds for tendon and ligament repair why is prestressing important? Foot Ankle Spec 2009;2(1):51–2.
26. O'Brien WR, Friederich NF, Muller W. The effects of stress relaxation on initial graft loads during anterior cruciate ligament reconstruction. Orthop Trans 1989;13:316–7.
27. Graf BK, Vanderby R, Ulm MJ, et al. Effect of preconditioning on the viscoelastic response of primate patellar tendon. Arthroscopy 1994;10:90–6.
28. Rogell MR, Parks BG, O'Donnell JB. Soaking versus moist storage of autologous patellar tendon before implantation for ACL reconstruction: a cadaver study. Orthopedics 2008;31:1194.
29. Lee MS. GraftJacket augmentation of chronic Achilles tendon ruptures. Orthopedics 2004;27:S151–3.
30. Lee DK. Achilles tendon repair with acellular tissue graft augmentation in neglected ruptures. J Foot Ankle Surg 2007;46(6):451–5.
31. Brigido SA, Schwartz E, Barnett L, et al. Reconstruction of the diseased Achilles tendon using an acellular human dermal graft followed by early mobilization a preliminary series. Tech Foot Ankle Surg 2007;6(4):249–53.
32. Lee DK. A preliminary study on the effects of acellular tissue graft augmentation in acute Achilles tendon ruptures. J Foot Ankle Surg 2008;47(1):8–12.
33. Lee DK. Effects of posterior tibial tendon augmented with biografts and calcaneal osteotomy in stage II adult-acquired flatfoot deformity. Foot Ankle Spec 2009; 2(1):27–31.
34. Wren TA, Yerby SA, Beaupre GS, et al. Mechanical properties of the human Achilles tendon. Clin Biomech (Bristol, Avon) 2001;16(3):245–51.
35. Rubin L, Schweitzer S. The use of acellular biologic tissue patches in foot and ankle surgery. Clin Podiatr Med Surg 2005;22:533–52.
36. Hambley E. Recurrent dislocation of ankle due to rupture of external lateral ligament. Br Med J 1945;1:413.
37. Storen H. A new method for operative treatment of insufficiency of the lateral ligaments of the ankle joint. Acta Chir Scand 1959;117:501–9.
38. Elmslie RC. Recurrent dislocation of the ankle joint. Ann Surg 1934;100:364–7.
39. Gschwend N. Lesions of the fibular ligaments: a frequently unrecognized result of sprain of the foot. Praxis 1958;47(35):809–12.
40. Weber BG, Hupfauer W. On the treatment of freshly ruptured ibular collateral ligaments and chronic insufficiency of the fibular collateral ligaments. Arch Orthop Unfallchir 1969;65(3):251–7.
41. Brostrom L. Sprained ankles III. Clinical observations in recent ligament ruptures. Acta Chir Scand 1965;130:560–9.
42. Sullivan EK, Kamstock DA, Turner AS, et al. Evaluation of a flexible collagen surgical patch for reinforcement of a fascial defect: experimental study in a sheep model. J Biomed Mater Res B Appl Biomater 2008;87(1):88–94.

Augmentation of Atrophic Plantar Soft Tissue with an Acellular Dermal Allograft: A Series Review

Thomas M. Rocchio, DPM[a,b,c],*

KEYWORDS

- Fat pad augmentation • Minimally invasive
- Parachute technique • Graftjacket • Plantar foot

Pain on the plantar aspect of the foot during weight bearing is a common result of atrophy of the fat pad. Age-related biomechanical property changes of the fat pad tissue may be associated with a higher incidence of foot pain and injury in the elderly.[1–3] The plantar fat pad may also become displaced, destroyed, or atrophied through traumatic events, such as repeated steroid injections, osseous fractures, sports injuries, burns, scarring from surgical incisions, or lengthy periods of weight bearing, especially in the presence of an orthopedic deformity.[4,5] Atrophy, displacement, or destruction of the plantar fat pad decreases the shock absorption quality and capabilities of the foot, leading to pain from increasing force placed on local anatomic structures. Increased pressure to underlying bone and soft tissue structures from fat pad degradation can result in subcalcaneal spurs, pain, capsulitis, painful callus, or ulceration.[2,3,6–8]

Over the past several decades, many surgical procedures have been presented, intending to restore, replenish, or augment atrophied fat pad thickness when conservative management has not produced satisfactory results.[2,9] Surgical treatments have included plantar soft tissue repositioning, autolipotransplantation, and injections of synthetic and bioengineered products. To date, the medical community has not adopted a single treatment method, because sufficient corroborating clinical evidence has not been reported to merit a standard of care procedure. The chief complaint with many of these techniques has been the lack of sustained tissue thickness over

Financial Disclosure Obligation: Thomas M. Rocchio, DPM, is a consultant for Wright Medical Technology, Inc.

[a] PA Podiatry, Allentown, PA 18104, USA
[b] PA Foot and Ankle Associates, 2200 West Hamilton Street, Suite 308, Allentown, PA 18104, USA
[c] Easton Hospital Wound Healing Center, Easton, PA 18040, USA
* Corresponding author.
E-mail address: contact@pafeet.com

Clin Podiatr Med Surg 26 (2009) 545–557
doi:10.1016/j.cpm.2009.07.001
0891-8422/09/$ – see front matter © 2009 Elsevier Inc. All rights reserved.

time, requiring a reapplication of the treatment.[9] Plantar soft tissue repositioning, although intrinsically offering an autologous tissue bulking option, is not a favored surgical option, because of the morbidity at the host site, the invasive nature of the procedure, and the higher risk of painful plantar scarring. Synthetic, autologous, and bioengineered tissue supplements have been investigated for fat pad augmentation, based on material success in non–weight-bearing areas of the body, such as the face.[10–12] Although there have been reports of positive results in these non–weight-bearing applications, reapplication may still be required.[13–16] It has been theorized that supplementation for plantar soft tissue applications may not produce long-term correction and pain relief, because of the migration tendencies that come with increased weight bearing, overall treatment volume, short resorption profile, or inconsistent delivery of the supplementing materials.

The purpose of this article is to provide a retrospective review of the results of a consecutive series of patients treated for fat pad atrophy of the plantar foot, using a minimally invasive implantation of an acellular human dermal allograft (Graftjacket Regenerative Tissue Matrix, Wright Medical Technology, Inc, Arlington, TN, USA) as a tissue augmentation. This material was chosen for the fat pad supplementation because of previous reports of success in tendon and ligament augmentation,[17–21] wound healing,[22–25] and interpositional arthroplasty.[26,27]

MATERIALS AND METHODS

A consecutive series of patients whose atrophy of the fat pad was surgically treated using a minimally invasive "parachute technique," with an acellular human dermal allograft as the augmenting material, was reviewed. Patient records were evaluated for demographic information, amount of graft used, operative site, additional procedures, comorbidities, ultrasound measurements, length of follow-up, complications, and patient satisfaction. Diagnostic ultrasound measurements were taken at time periods of 1, 3, 6, and 12 months, as appropriate. Patient satisfaction was determined at the last postoperative follow-up, using a verbal patient satisfaction classification. A total of 25 patients (26 treatments) were evaluated, following fat pad augmentation surgery.

Patient Selection and Preoperative Protocol

All patients selected for this procedure presented with a history of plantar weight-bearing pain or ulceration that was nonresponsive to conservative treatments. This conservative treatment included off-loading, debridement of hyperkeratotic lesions, or wound care. Those with a deficit in the plantar soft tissue, as determined by diagnostic ultrasound examination, were considered for this procedure. In cases of orthopedic deformity, additional procedures were performed at the time of the fat pad augmentation.

All patients received full biomechanical examination, radiographic examination, and diagnostic ultrasound imaging (**Fig. 1**A, B) of the plantar soft tissue of the afflicted foot. This ultrasound imaging provided qualification of the deficit and quantification of the extent of atrophy. All patients had their normal value calculated, with comparison to an asymptomatic contralateral limb or an adjacent metatarsal's plantar soft tissue. Ultrasound measurements were used to map and determine the thickness and total area of the symptomatic deficit. The diagnostic ultrasound-mapped deficit was used to determine the appropriate size of the augmenting material needed for the procedure. Generally, the thickest acellular human dermal graft available (Graftjacket

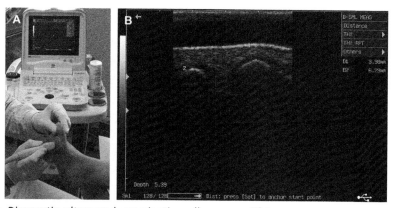

Fig. 1. Diagnostic ultrasound examination allows quantifying accurate measurement of deficit. (*A*) Measuring the metatarsal fat pad thickness. (*B*) Example of diagnostic ultrasound image of plantar fat pad at the level of the metatarsal head. Note the decreased soft tissue submetatarsal 2 compared with submetatarsal 3.

MaxForce *Extreme* Matrix, Wright Medical Technology, Inc, Arlington, TN, USA) was chosen, with an average thickness of 2 mm in a single sheet.

Surgical Technique

Incision planning focused on avoidance of the weight-bearing plantar skin, to help eliminate the complication of a painful plantar scar. This was especially important when patients had a history of ulceration or comorbidities, such as diabetes. The incision length varied, especially if accommodating concurrent osseous procedures. At the metatarsal level, the incision was a longitudinal medial for a submetatarsal 1 deficit, a longitudinal lateral for a submetatarsal 5 deficit, or a transverse sulcus for isolated deficits of submetatarsal 2 through 4. For the minimal incision parachute technique used here, the incision was roughly one-third of the length of the acellular dermal graft, but it was longer when accommodating significant increases in the thickness of the augmenting material. Once the incision was carried fully through the skin, blunt and sharp dissection was used to create a pocket in the deep subcutaneous tissue. This pocket was equivalent in size to the preoperative measurements of the fat pad deficit determined during the ultrasound (**Fig. 2**).

To prepare the acellular human dermal matrix for implantation, the matrix was soaked in a saline solution according to the manufacturer's instructions for use. After rehydration, the graft was measured, the size reverified according to the deficit determined, and the graft trimmed to the desired size. If the desired thickness was significantly more than the 2 mm graft, the graft was folded to the desired thickness or stacked with additional pieces of graft. In cases of deficits greater than 4 mm, the 2 mm thick acellular dermal graft was only stacked to 4 mm. In the author's experience, it was not necessary to augment the full thickness of the deficit to achieve pain relief and a satisfactory result. This was found to be the case in several surgically augmented patients with significantly larger plantar fat pad deficits than 4 mm, all resulting in full relief of pain with only 4 mm of augmentation graft thickness used. Use of a significantly larger thickness of augmentation would also require an increased incision, with a more difficult insertion predictability. The graft tissue was cut slightly larger than the preoperative measurements, to assure full area augmentation. Intraoperative

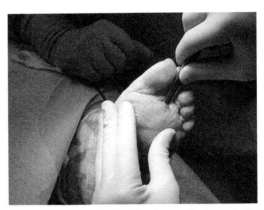

Fig. 2. Creation of the desired-size pocket in the deep soft tissue, following the skin markings made using the preoperative ultrasound measurements.

trimming of excess graft was easily accomplished, whereas adding to an undersized graft was not desirable (**Fig. 3**).

Using a method employed in plastic surgery for soft tissue augmentation, absorbable traction sutures were applied to the corners of the graft. This suture was also used to hold multiple pieces of graft tissue in cases that required graft stacking (**Fig. 4**). The sutures that were attached to each corner of the graft tissue were placed on a needle driver and driven from inside the surgically created pocket out through the designated corner. As the sutures were evenly and gently drawn, the graft tissue was inserted into the pocket through the incision; then the sutures were further uniformly drawn through the skin, to evenly and reproducibly open the graft tissue like a parachute, until it lay flat in the pocket (**Fig. 5**).

For a full incisional approach, a nonabsorbable double-needled suture was used. An open loop with ends about 3 mm apart was placed in each of the deep designated corners of the graft. With this technique, a knot was not used to secure the suture in the graft material (**Fig. 6**). Through the retracted pocket opening, the 2 needles from the deep distal and the 2 needles from the deep proximal graft sutures were driven from inside the pocket through the skin. The 2 needles from each corner exited

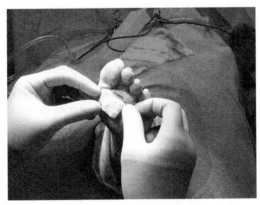

Fig. 3. Intraoperative graft sizing against the measured external skin markings.

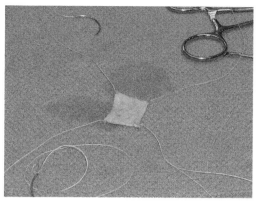

Fig. 4. Desired-size graft with absorbable suture tied to each of the 4 corners of the graft. These sutures also hold staked graft pieces together if thicker augmentation is desired.

the skin approximately 3 mm apart. The traction sutures were then used to draw the graft material into the pocket gently and evenly (**Fig. 7**).

Using this parachute technique, the acellular human dermal matrix was uniformly positioned in the pocket. If excess graft was apparent, it was trimmed as necessary. Once positioned, the deep corner suture ends were tied together outside the skin. External knotting secured the graft until appropriate incorporation was achieved. When the sutures were removed, no suture material remained in the patient, because internal knots were not used to secure the graft (**Fig. 8**). For the minimal incision approach, the absorbable sutures were tied over a centrally located folded gauze to hold the graft in place and provide a light pressure dressing.

Postoperative Protocol

Patients were not allowed to bear weight for the first 2 postoperative weeks. Absorbable sutures were cut flush with the skin at the 1- to 2-week postoperative period (**Fig. 9**A, B). If no additional procedures were performed, weight bearing was allowed after this 2-week period. If additional osseous or soft tissue procedures were

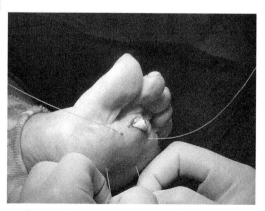

Fig. 5. After the suture from each of the 4 corners of the graft are driven from inside the pocket through the skin in each of the 4 designated corners of the pocket, the graft is gently drawn into the pocket, opened, and fixed with these traction sutures.

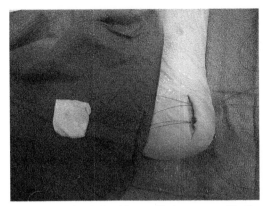

Fig. 6. Cadaver model showing the 2 double-needled sutures with the needles from each designated corner exiting approximately 3 mm apart from the deep corners of the pocket (out of view). Note the loops in what will be the 2 deep corners of the graft tissue. This suture will facilitate insertion of the graft and then act to anchor the graft in the created surgical pocket.

performed, the postoperative course was determined by the longest healing procedure. Diagnostic ultrasound examinations were repeated at the 1-, 3-, and 6-month postoperative periods, with several patients undergoing 1-year ultrasound examination.

RESULTS

In this retrospective consecutive series, 26 fat pad surgical treatments were performed in 25 patients between September 2005 and December 2008, using this technique. The population consisted of 5 men and 20 women, with an average age of 51.2 years (range, 34–72 years) at the time of surgery. The surgical site treated was the lateral plantar midfoot fat pad in 1 case, heel fat pad in 3 cases, and submetatarsal fat pad in the remaining 22 cases. In 5 instances, patients had comorbidities of diabetes, and 4 of these patients had previous diabetic foot ulcers, 3 of whom had

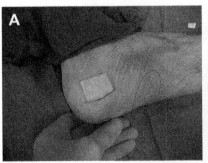
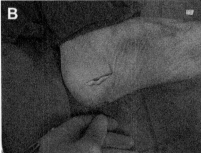

Fig. 7. (*A*) As the sutures are evenly and gently drawn, the graft tissue is inserted into the surgically created pocket. This technique can be duplicated with any augmentation procedure with confidence of a predictable and even application of the graft. (*B*) The graft is inserted and the sutures are tied to secure the graft. On suture removal, there will be no retained suture material, as no knots were needed in the pocket.

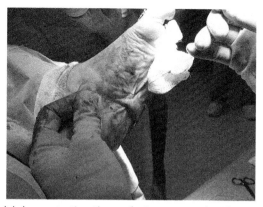

Fig. 8. Cadaver model demonstrating the graft tissue secured with 2 external knots. When these sutures are removed in the postoperative period, there will be no retained suture in the patient.

ulceration at the time of the fat pad augmentation. The average approximate thickness of acellular human dermal matrix used was 2.7 mm, with 2 mm used in 17 cases and 4 mm used in 9 cases. Of the 26 cases, 13 were performed with additional procedures: 8 cases of dorsal displacement metatarsal osteotomy; 2 cases of plantar metatarsal condylectomy; and 3 cases of plantar exostectomy and ulceration excisional debridement, with acellular dermal skin grafting.

The average postoperative follow-up for this series was 6 months (range, 1–27 months). Of the 26 cases, 11 were released from care, 7 were lost to follow-up, and 8 continue to be followed up. The average follow-up time for patients released from care was 8 months (range, 3–27 months); for those lost to follow-up, 2.9 months (range, 1–6 months); and for those actively being followed up, 5.9 months (range, 3–15 months). All patients provided a satisfaction level at their last postoperative visit. The average patient satisfaction for the population was 95.8%. All 22 nondiabetic sensate patients related postoperative pain relief, with 20 patients relating 100% pain relief at their final postoperative visit; 1 patient, 80%, after the 3-month visit, and 1 patient, 40%, with continued pain 1 year after the procedure. All 4 diabetic patients had a high degree of neuropathy preoperatively, and have gone on to full healing postoperatively, with no

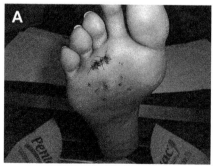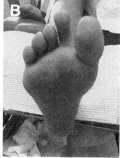

Fig. 9. (*A*) 1 week after surgery. Note the surgical pen marks forming a box that shows the size of the graft area. These markings are where each of the 4 traction sutures exited the pocket. Note that the minimal incision is one-third the width of the graft. (*B*) 4 months after surgery. Notice the resolution of the sub–fourth-metatarsal intractable plantar keratosis.

recurrence of ulceration to date. **Fig. 10** shows the average ultrasound preoperative fat pad measurement and those at postoperative 1-month, 3-month, 6-month, and 12-month time points. Measurements were not taken for all patients at all time points because of their different follow-up times, the diagnostic learning curve, and modality availability in the clinical setting. Within this series, all patients had preoperative measurements, 23 had 1-month measurements; 17, 3-month; 9, 6-month; and 2, 12-month. **Fig. 11** shows the average percentage of thickness retained after the first postoperative measurement. No complications were observed with this procedure intraoperatively. Postoperatively, 1 patient had a mild infection, with incision dehiscence at the implantation entry site. This was a diabetic man who had adjunct procedures performed, specifically, ulceration debridement and grafting and heel exostectomy. This patient responded well to oral antibiotics and healed the dehiscence through secondary intention, without the need to return to the operating room. This diabetic man also had a 3-year preoperative history of recurrent plantar heel ulceration. Ulceration has not recurred 1 year after the operation.

DISCUSSION

Historically, plantar fat pad augmentation techniques have a range of short-term success; the greatest disadvantage of these procedures is the inability to maintain the desired thickness correction, because of product breakdown, absorption, or migration. This results in a recurrence of pain and necessitates additional augmentation procedures to maintain an acceptable correction. Injectable treatments, synthetic or natural in origin, have been of primary interest in plantar fat pad augmentation, because of their ease of application and minimally invasive technique.

Injectable silicone investigations have generated many reports; however, much of the information regarding injectable silicone use in the plantar fat pad stems from a single institution and, although supplied over a long period, is anecdotal in nature. Balkin[28] reported on his 41-year use of injectable silicone for foot applications in more than 1500 patients. In his practice, a series of approximately 4 injections was required to achieve initial reduction in pain. Long-term follow-up indicated that 60%

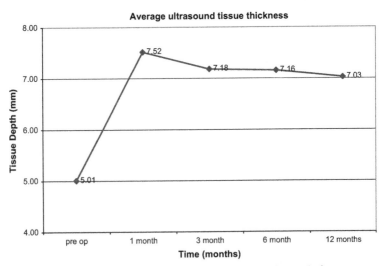

Fig. 10. Average ultrasound measurements over set postoperative periods.

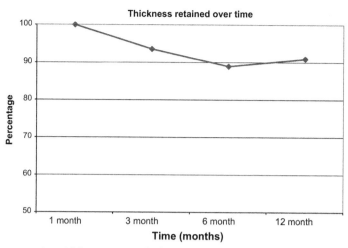

Fig. 11. Augmentation thickness retained after the first postoperative visit.

to 80% experienced moderate-to-complete pain relief. Approximately 50% of those treated required 1 or more reapplications in the following 1 to 20 years.[28] Local fluid migration was seen if large quantities of silicone were used or the area was overinjected. In some instances, these overinjected areas merited surgical removal. There were also instances when skin discoloration occurred.[28] In a randomized controlled trial comparing injectable silicone with a placebo treatment, at 3-, 6-, 12- and 24-month follow-up, injectable silicone treatments increased the plantar tissue thickness and decreased the peak plantar pressure at the 12-month time point.[8,29] Reduction of the plantar tissue augmentation was seen in the early postoperative time points, indicating some migration of the silicone away from the weight-bearing area.[29] At 24 months, the plantar tissue thickness was still improved; however, there was no difference in the plantar pressure from baseline. Over time, a reduction in the volume of plantar thickness was seen and the cushioning effect of the injectable silicone decreased, indicating that more injections would be necessary to maintain the effects of the treatment.[29] In the randomized trial, ulcers at the injection sites were the primary complication seen over time.[29] A histologic study, by Wallace and colleagues,[30] analyzed biopsies from patients treated with injectable silicone over a 38-year time period. They grouped specimens according to the time in vivo, to determine differences in response and appearance of the material over time. The host response to the liquid silicone was initially characterized by histiocytic phagocytosis of the liquid silicone by an abundance of macrophages. Over time, the size of the silicone droplets within the samples was reduced and an increased appearance of "necrotic Swiss cheese–like fibrosis" was seen. The silicone was phagocytized by histiocytes over time and migratory particles were found within macrophage vacuoles. The necrotic fibrosis did not seem to break down with increased implant longevity and was not associated with a host reaction. It was hypothesized that the mechanical pump action of ambulation was responsible for the changes in silicone droplet size over time and for local silicone fluid migration.[30] There were limited instances of foreign-body giant cells and asteroid bodies. Silicone treatments in facial applications have also been reported as causing complications, such as nodules, migration, infection, and granulomas.[31,32] Even in non–weight-bearing applications, liquid silicone may require reapplication or may offer asymmetrical or inconsistent augmentation.[32]

Autologous fat has been readily advocated as a filler for depressed areas of the face.[11,15] Due to the short duration of benefit, aesthetic results, and degree of variability of autologous fat, a multitude of alternative fillers have been investigated in non–weight-bearing areas such as the face.[11,15,16] These fillers are used in the aging face and in HIV-associated lipodystrophy.[11,15,33] Alternative fillers to silicone and autologous fat have included poly-L-lactic acid (PLA); collagen; hyaluronic acid; hydrogel (Bio-Alcamid [Polymekon, Srl, Brindisi, Italy]); polyvinyl alcohol; calcium hydroxylapatite; polymethyl methacrylate; and polyacrylamide gel.[10–12,33] Biodegradable fillers, such as PLA and hyaluronic acid, require multiple applications in these non–weight-bearing areas, with possible reapplication over time due to a lower life span.[11,13,33] Complications have been reported, such as subcutaneous noninflammatory nodules,[33] granulomas,[12,34] migration, inflammatory nodules, allergic reactions, and vascular occlusions.[12,16,32]

Autolipotransplantation has also been used in the lower extremity, for cosmetic results and fat pad atrophy.[9,14] In lower limb circumferential atrophy applications, it has shown positive results; however, fat resorption is often required, needing overcorrection or multiple applications.[14] In 1994, Chairman's[9] review of 50 patients, treated with autolipotransplantation for fat pad atrophy, also highlighted this loss of correction over time. In this technique, suctioned fat from other areas of the body was injected, in a fanlike fashion, into the subcutaneous space within the fat pad region. Although all patients reported initial pain relief, the transferred suctioned fat only maintained 32% of its volume and 41% of its thickness, with 2 of the 50 patients having 100% resorption of the autolipotransplantation.[9]

These applications indicate that loss of correction and material resorption constitute the greatest shortcomings of many augmenting materials. Other problems encountered in non–weight-bearing applications that are of greater concern in pressurized areas, such as the atrophic fat pad, are inconsistent delivery, difficulty in controlling the placement, and local migration of the augmenting material. The ideal tissue filler would retain its physical properties, would be easily manipulated, easily obtained, inexpensive, and effective, and would offer predictable short- and long-term results.[31]

Our goal, in using this minimally invasive parachute technique, was to provide a graft that would be repopulated by noninflammatory host cells, would incorporate easily into the surrounding tissue without being resorbed, and would maintain consistent properties and dimensions over time. Preclinical and clinical reports have revealed these attributes in the acellular human dermal matrix chosen, including in applications such as wound healing,[24,25,35] tendon augmentation,[18–20,36–39] and facial soft tissue augmentation.[40,41] Preclinical animal studies, in rat,[42,43] canine,[44] and porcine models,[43] have consistently shown that this material is repopulated by host cells, revascularizes over time, incorporates into the surrounding tissue through a regenerative healing process, and does not elicit an inflammatory response.[42–45] As seen in animal models, graft incorporation and graft transition to the surrounding tissue type have been confirmed in a clinical instance of graft biopsy of the Achilles tendon.[46]

Unlike injectable materials, the thickness, length, and width of the acellular human dermal matrix are predetermined during preoperative measurement. The extent of tissue thickening and the placement of the graft will not diminish with initial postoperative massage or pressure. Using the minimally invasive parachute technique, the material is secured in the deep soft tissue and is allowed to stabilize during the first 2 postoperative weeks. As this matrix becomes incorporated into the surrounding host tissue, future surgical interventions would not be prevented or interrupted by the presence of this augmentation. As seen in this series, with this technique, there is little loss of original correction at the 6-month and 1-year postaugmentation time points. This method is reproducible and offers consistent patient satisfaction over time.

Although the parachute technique uses minimal incision, it is more invasive than an injection augmentation that uses a flowable substance such as silicone. With incision and dissection, there is risk of neurovascular damage and painful scar formation. Although the parachute technique is not technically demanding, it is easy to perform incomplete dissection of the deep subcutaneous pocket. This failure to eliminate all fibrous septa from this surgically created pocket will lead to a bunching up of the graft material with inconsistent placement.

SUMMARY

Treatment of plantar fat pad migration and atrophy has been a concern for physicians and surgeons for decades. Patients can present with pain, callus formation, or ulceration.

The data collected over 10 years on acellular dermal graft use in other areas of the body, and the results of the subjects in this study, support the author's opinion that the "parachute technique" for plantar fat pad augmentation solves the problem practically and permanently. The minimal incision approach of the parachute technique has allowed a more aggressive treatment of patients with significant comorbidities. The most significant high-risk group to benefit from this procedure has been the diabetic population with a history of ulceration.

This study had patients with varied presentation, including plantar soft tissue deficits, such as a tissue-destroying burn with a skin graft over the plantar metatarsal capsule, a simple painful intractable plantar keratosis, and neuropathic ulcerations in the diabetic foot. Early in the study, these higher-risk patients with comorbidities, such as diabetes, were excluded. Their inclusion later in the study helped to demonstrate the strength and safety of this procedure in this more diverse group.

REFERENCES

1. Hsu TC, Wang CL, Tsai WC, et al. Comparison of the mechanical properties of the heel pad between young and elderly adults. Arch Phys Med Rehabil 1998;79(9): 1101–4.
2. Ozdemir H, Soyuncu Y, Ozgorgen M, et al. Effects of changes in heel fat pad thickness and elasticity on heel pain. J Am Podiatr Med Assoc 2004;94(1):47–52.
3. Hsu TC, Wang CL, Shau YW, et al. Altered heel-pad mechanical properties in patients with type 2 diabetes mellitus. Diabet Med 2000;17(12):854–9.
4. Basadonna PT, Rucco V, Gasparini D, et al. Plantar fat pad atrophy after corticosteroid injection for an interdigital neuroma: a case report. Am J Phys Med Rehabil 1999;78(3):283–5.
5. Aldridge T. Diagnosing heel pain in adults. Am Fam Physician 2004;70(2):332–8.
6. Cheung YY, Doyley M, Miller TB, et al. Magnetic resonance elastography of the plantar fat pads: preliminary study in diabetic patients and asymptomatic volunteers. J Comput Assist Tomogr 2006;30(2):321–6.
7. Turgut A, Gokturk E, Kose N, et al. The relationship of heel pad elasticity and plantar heel pain. Clin Orthop Relat Res 1999;(360):191–6.
8. van Schie CH, Whalley A, Vileikyte L, et al. Efficacy of injected liquid silicone in the diabetic foot to reduce risk factors for ulceration: a randomized double-blind placebo-controlled trial. Diabetes Care 2000;23(5):634–8.
9. Chairman EL. Restoration of the plantar fat pad with autolipotransplantation. J Foot Ankle Surg 1994;33(4):373–9.

10. Honig J. Cheek augmentation with Bio-Alcamid in facial lipoatrophy in HIV sero-positive patients. J Craniofac Surg 2008;19(4):1085–8.
11. Bucky LP, Kanchwala SK. The role of autologous fat and alternative fillers in the aging face. Plast Reconstr Surg 2007;120(Suppl 6):89S–97S.
12. Vedamurthy M. Standard guidelines for the use of dermal fillers. Indian J Dermatol Venereol Leprol 2008;74(Suppl):S23–7.
13. Mallewa JE, Wilkins E, Vilar J, et al. HIV-associated lipodystrophy: a review of underlying mechanisms and therapeutic options. J Antimicrob Chemother 2008;62(4):648–60.
14. Mojallal A, Veber M, Shipkov C, et al. Analysis of a series of autologous fat tissue transfer for lower limb atrophies. Ann Plast Surg 2008;61(5):537–43.
15. Orlando G, Guaraldi G, De Fazio D, et al. Long-term psychometric outcomes of facial lipoatrophy therapy: forty-eight-week observational, nonrandomized study. AIDS Patient Care STDS 2007;21(11):833–42.
16. Smith KC. Reversible vs. nonreversible fillers in facial aesthetics: concerns and considerations [abstract]. Dermatol Online J 2008 Aug 15;14(8):3.
17. Rizio L, Jarmon N. Chronic quadriceps rupture: treatment with lengthening and early mobilization without cerclage augmentation and a report of three cases. J Knee Surg 2008;21(1):34–8.
18. Lee DK. Achilles tendon repair with acellular tissue graft augmentation in neglected ruptures. J Foot Ankle Surg 2007;46(6):451–5.
19. Lee DK. A preliminary study on the effects of acellular tissue graft augmentation in acute Achilles tendon ruptures. J Foot Ankle Surg 2008;47(1):8–12.
20. Brigido SA, Schwartz E, Barnett L, et al. Reconstruction of the diseased Achilles tendon using an acellular human dermal graft followed by early mobilization-a preliminary series. Tech Foot Ankle Surg 2007;6(4):249–53.
21. Furukawa K, Pichora J, Steinmann S, et al. Efficacy of interference screw and double-docking methods using palmaris longus and GraftJacket for medial collateral ligament reconstruction of the elbow. J Shoulder Elbow Surg 2007; 16(4):449–53.
22. Winters CL, Brigido SA, Liden BA, et al. A multicenter study involving the use of a human acellular dermal regenerative tissue matrix for the treatment of diabetic lower extremity wounds. Adv Skin Wound Care 2008;21(8):375–81.
23. Randall KL, Booth BA, Miller AJ, et al. Use of an acellular regenerative tissue matrix in combination with vacuum-assisted closure therapy for treatment of a diabetic foot wound. J Foot Ankle Surg 2008;47(5):430–3.
24. Brigido SA. The use of an acellular dermal regenerative tissue matrix in the treatment of lower extremity wounds: a prospective 16-week pilot study. Int Wound J 2006;3(3):181–7.
25. Martin BR, Sangalang M, Wu S, et al. Outcomes of allogenic acellular matrix therapy in treatment of diabetic foot wounds: an initial experience. Int Wound J 2005;2(2):161–5.
26. Berlet G, Hyer C, Lee T, et al. A soft-tissue interpositional arthroplasty technique of the first metatarsophalangeal joint for the treatment of advanced hallux rigidus using a human acellular dermal regenerative tissue matrix. Tech Foot Ankle Surg 2006;5(4):257–65.
27. Berlet GC, Hyer CF, Lee TH, et al. Interpositional arthroplasty of the first MTP joint using a regenerative tissue matrix for the treatment of advanced hallux rigidus. Foot Ankle Int 2008;29(1):10–21.
28. Balkin SW. Injectable silicone and the foot: a 41-year clinical and histologic history. Dermatol Surg 2005;31(11 Pt 2):1555–9 [discussion: 1560].

29. van Schie CH, Whalley A, Armstrong DG, et al. The effect of silicone injections in the diabetic foot on peak plantar pressure and plantar tissue thickness: a 2-year follow-up. Arch Phys Med Rehabil 2002;83(7):919–23.
30. Wallace WD, Balkin SW, Kaplan L, et al. The histologic host response to liquid silicone injections for prevention of pressure-related ulcers of the foot: a 38-year study. J Am Podiatr Med Assoc 2004;94(6):550–7.
31. Anastassov GE, Schulhof S, Lumerman H. Complications after facial contour augmentation with injectable silicone. Diagnosis and treatment. Report of a severe case. Int J Oral Maxillofac Surg 2008;37(10):955–60.
32. Duffy DM. Liquid silicone for soft tissue augmentation. Dermatol Surg 2005;31(11 Pt 2):1530–41.
33. Carey DL, Baker D, Rogers GD, et al. A randomized, multicenter, open-label study of poly-L-lactic acid for HIV-1 facial lipoatrophy. J Acquir Immune Defic Syndr 2007;46(5):581–9.
34. Stewart DB, Morganroth GS, Mooney MA, et al. Management of visible granulomas following periorbital injection of poly-L-lactic acid. Ophthal Plast Reconstr Surg 2007;23(4):298–301.
35. Brigido SA, Boc SF, Lopez RC. Effective management of major lower extremity wounds using an acellular regenerative tissue matrix: a pilot study. Orthopedics 2004;27(Suppl 1):s145–9.
36. Burkhead W, Schiffern S, Krishnan S. Use of graft jacket as an augmentation for massive rotator cuff tears. Semin Arthroplasty 2007;18:11–8.
37. Labbe MR. Arthroscopic technique for patch augmentation of rotator cuff repairs. Arthroscopy 2006;22(10):1136, e1131–e1136.
38. Snyder S, Bond J. Technique for arthroscopic replacement of severely damaged rotator cuff using "Graftjacket" allograft. Oper Tech Sports Med 2007;15:86–94.
39. Bond JL, Dopirak RM, Higgins J, et al. Arthroscopic replacement of massive, irreparable rotator cuff tears using a GraftJacket allograft: technique and preliminary results. Arthroscopy 2008;24(4):403–9, e401.
40. Shorr N, Perry JD, Goldberg RA, et al. The safety and applications of acellular human dermal allograft in ophthalmic plastic and reconstructive surgery: a preliminary report. Ophthal Plast Reconstr Surg 2000;16(3):223–30.
41. Costantino PD, Govindaraj S, Hiltzik DH, et al. Acellular dermis for facial soft tissue augmentation: preliminary report. Arch Facial Plast Surg 2001;3(1):38–43.
42. Turner A, Blum B, Burgess A. Effects of acellular human dermal matrix thickness in cellular repopulation capabilities in a submuscular rat model. Paper presented at American College of Foot and Ankle Surgeons; Long Beach (CA), 2008.
43. Beniker D, McQuillan D, Livesey S, et al. The use of acellular dermal matrix as a scaffold for periosteum replacement. Orthopedics 2003;26(Suppl 5):s591–6.
44. Adams JE, Zobitz ME, Reach JS Jr, et al. Rotator cuff repair using an acellular dermal matrix graft: an in vivo study in a canine model. Arthroscopy 2006; 22(7):700–9.
45. Harper J, McQuillan D. A novel regenerative tissue matrix (RTM) technology for connective tissue reconstruction. Wounds 2007;19(6):163–8.
46. Liden BA, Simmons M. Histologic evaluation of a 6-month GraftJacket matrix biopsy used for Achilles tendon augmentation. J Am Podiatr Med Assoc 2009; 99(2):104–7.

Bone and Wound Healing Augmentation with Platelet-Rich Plasma

Simon E. Smith, BPod, MPod, FACPS[a,b,]*, Thomas S. Roukis, DPM, PhD, FACFAS[c]

KEYWORDS

- Autologous platelet-rich plasma
- Autologous platelet-poor plasma
- Bone graft • Wound coverage • Ulceration

Orthobiologics is one of the largest growing sectors within the medical device industry. Historically, orthobiologics in orthopedic surgery has encompassed technologies, such as bone graft substitutes and resorbable fixation; however, the use of autologous platelet-rich plasma (PRP) for the facilitation and modulation of bone and soft tissue healing has generated much interest in the fields of reconstructive plastic surgery, spine surgery, oral and maxillofacial surgery, and advanced wound care. PRP is defined as a sequestration and concentration of platelets within the plasma fraction of autologous blood.

Investigations into the efficacy of PRP and its clinical use have emerged from the greater understanding of bone and soft tissue healing at a cellular level. Components within blood constituents, such as cytokines and growth factors derived from platelets, are integral to the initiation and modulation of the healing process. The concept that these growth factors can be concentrated, such as with the production of PRP, and applied in a therapeutic manner to alter or accelerate tissue healing is both plausible and compelling, and warrants further investigation. This article presents the biology, background, and evidence for the use of PRP.

Disclaimer: The opinions or assertions contained herein are the private view of the author and are not to be construed as official or reflecting the views of the Department of the Army or the Department of Defense.
[a] Australasian College of Podiatric Surgeons, Australia
[b] Musculoskeletal Research Center & Department of Podiatry, La Trobe University, Kingsbury Drive, Bundoora, VIC, Australia 3086
[c] Limb Preservation Service and Director, Limb Preservation Complex Lower Extremity Surgery and Research Fellowship, Vascular/Endovascular Surgery Service, Department of Surgery, Madigan Army Medical Center, 9040-A Fitzsimmons Avenue, MCHJ-SV, Tacoma, WA 98431, USA
* Corresponding author. Musculoskeletal Research Center, Department of Podiatry, La Trobe University, Kingsbury Drive, Bundoora, VIC, Australia 3086.
E-mail address: simonsmithpod@optusnet.com.au (S.E. Smith).

Clin Podiatr Med Surg 26 (2009) 559–588
doi:10.1016/j.cpm.2009.07.002
0891-8422/09/$ – see front matter
© 2009 Elsevier Inc. All rights reserved.
podiatric.theclinics.com

PLATELET BIOLOGY AND HEMOSTASIS

Platelets are colorless cell fragments, produced when the cytoplasm of bone marrow cells, termed megakaryocytes, fragment, and enter the circulation.[1] However, megakaryocytes have been identified in intravascular sites within the lung, leading to a theory that platelets are formed from their parent cell in the pulmonary circulation.[2] Platelets cannot replicate, thus the life span of a platelet is 5 to 9 days, at which time they are removed from the bloodstream by macrophages.[3] They primarily reside in the intravascular space, with approximately 25% existing in the liver and spleen.[4] Platelets are approximately 3.0 by 0.5 μm in diameter and are characteristically discoid in shape.[2,5] They are without a nucleus, but contain organelles such as mitochondria and granules (α, δ, and λ), with α granules containing more than 30 bioactive proteins that have a pivotal role in hemostasis and hard and soft tissue healing.[5] Each platelet has approximately 50 to 80 α granules.[5] Platelet counts of 150,000 to 400,000 mm^3 within the human blood stream are considered normal.[4]

Platelets ordinarily do not interact with other platelets or other cell types, unless they are exposed to a stimulatory agonist.[6] After tissue injury, cellular membranes release thromboxane A$_2$ and prostaglandin 2α, leading to initial vasoconstriction.[7] Circulating platelets are exposed directly to subendothelial matrix proteins, such as collagen, von Willebrand factor, fibronectin, thrombospondin-1, and laminins.[6,8,9] The net result is adhesion of platelets and initial thrombus formation, followed by aggregation of platelets at the respective site.[9] This process is called *activation*, which includes a change in platelet morphology with the manifestation of pseudopodia and granular release.[1,10]

One of the most rapidly secreted substances from platelets is adenosine diphosphate, which is also released from injured vascular cells and red blood cells. It is a potent agonist for platelet aggregation.[6] Furthermore, the passive release of serotonin and thromboxane from platelets further amplifies platelet activation.[6] Thrombin is also a strong agonist for platelet activation and granular secretion, as is epinephrine to a lesser extent.[6]

During the activation phase, α granules bind with the platelet plasma membrane and release their contents into the surroundings.[1,6,10]

The numerous peptides and proteins released from α granules (eg, growth factors, cytokines, and chemokines) aid in cellular migration and growth and include platelet-derived growth factor (PDGF), transforming growth factor (TGF)-β, insulin-like growth factor (IGF), vascular endothelial growth factor (VEGF), epidermal growth factor (EGF), platelet factor 4, interleukin (IL)-1, platelet-derived angiogenesis factor, platelet-derived endothelial growth factor, epithelial cell growth factor, osteocalcin, osteonectin, fibrinogen, vitronectin, fibronectin, and thrombospondin.[5,8,11–14]

Approximately 10 minutes after platelet aggregation/clotting, platelets begin to actively secrete these proteins to the extent that within 1 hour, approximately 95% of the α granule contents have been secreted.[11]

The progression of blood clotting follows the generation of thrombin and fibrin through the intrinsic and extrinsic pathways around the original platelet plug.[15] The intrinsic pathway is manifest from components solely within blood, and the extrinsic pathway requires cellular elements outside of the blood. The terminal cascade of interactions between cofactors and enzymes that result in a stable clot is the same for both pathways.

Platelets are involved in a multitude of steps during the propagation of a stable clot, consisting of fibrin, platelet aggregation, and red and white blood cells. During this formal clot maturation is when α granule contents are released, with the fibrin matrix acting as a reservoir of growth factors and proteins released from the enmeshed platelets. This initial activity of protein release is followed by the active synthesis and secretion of additional proteins by the platelet for the remainder of its life span (5–9 days).[11,16]

PLATELET ROLE IN WOUND HEALING

Platelets play a pivotal role in wound healing, principally through the generation and release of large quantities of growth factors. Once released from the α granules, the active growth factors bind to transmembrane receptors of target cells, such as mesenchymal stem cells, osteoblasts, fibroblasts, endothelial cells, and epidermal cells.[11] Platelet-derived factors directly influence cellular growth, morphogenesis, and differentiation. The growth factors released from α granules and their biologic activity are detailed later.

PLATELET-DERIVED GROWTH FACTOR

PDGF is a protein consisting of two subunits, α and β, and exists as PDGF-αα, PDGF-ββ, and PDGF-αβ.[17] PDGF is a powerful chemotactic agent for monocytes, neutrophils, smooth muscle cells, fibroblasts, mesenchymal stem cells, and osteoblasts and is involved in all three phases of wound healing.[18–20] PDGF is also a powerful mitogen and attaches to transmembrane receptors on target cells, particularly fibroblasts, smooth muscle cells, and osteoblasts, and increases the number of mesenchymal stem, osteoprogenitor, and endothelial cells.[21,22] These cell lines are responsible for connective and bone tissue healing and angiogenesis within the wound.[21,23] Additionally, PDGF has been reported to stimulate fibroblasts to contract collagen matrices and facilitate the myofibroblast phenotype.[24]

PDGF activates macrophages to secrete their own growth factors, which in turn stimulates growth factor secretion from surrounding tissue under the influence of macrophage action.[11,20] PDGF has also been seen to augment macrophage-mediated tissue debridement and granulation tissue formation.[25] Furthermore, it helps collagen breakdown during the remodeling phase of wound healing through up-regulating matrix metalloproteinases.[26] Through up-regulating the production of IGF-1 and thrombospondin-1, PDGF also plays a role in reepithelialization after wounding, wherein IGF-1 increases keratinocyte motility and thrombospondin-1 delays proteolytic degradation.[27–29]

Although its effect on angiogenesis is weaker than fibrogen growth factor (FGF) and VEGF, the positive influence of PDGF on blood vessel maturation and its synergistic effect with tissue hypoxia to increase expression of VEGF in wounds has also been reported.[30–32]

The therapeutic potential of PDGF in wound repair was identified by Grotendorst and colleagues,[33] who showed increased DNA synthesis, collagen deposition, and influx of connective tissue cells at 2 weeks, with PDGF contained within dead-space chambers, compared with controls in a rat model. Others have reported that recombinant PDGF-ββ, in supraphysiologic concentrations, transiently increases the acute inflammatory phase of wound healing. This effect results in acceleration of normal wound repair processes and early matrix deposition, which sustains a positive influence on wound healing.[18,33–42] PDGF-ββ was also observed to reverse deficient repair and restore normal tissue repair rates in surface radiation, ischemic- and diabetic-impaired wound healing, and ulceration.[41–54]

PDGF has been identified at fracture sites in humans.[55] Furthermore, PDGF has been observed to increase ectopic bone formation and alkaline phosphatase activity using demineralized bone matrix as a carrier in rats.[3] Tibial osteotomy sites in rabbits treated with PDGF impregnated within a collagen sponge show more advanced osteogenic differentiation and an increase in density and volume of callus compared with controls.[56]

TRANSFORMING GROWTH FACTOR β

TGF-β is a polypeptide and has five isoforms (TGF-β1–5). Platelets secrete isomers β1 and β2 and these factors are involved in all stages of wound healing, playing a role in inflammation, angiogenesis, reepithelialization, and connective tissue regeneration.[3] TGF-β stimulates monocytes to secrete growth factors (FGF, PDGF, IL-1, and TNF-α) and is chemotactic to macrophages, augmenting tissue debridement.[57,58] This factor also stimulates fibroblast chemotaxis and proliferation and is a potent stimulant for collagen synthesis, fibronectin, and proteoglycan synthesis from fibroblasts, protease inhibitors. It also influences the organization of extracellular matrix, scar remodeling, and contracture.[58–70] TGF-β is also involved in up-regulation of VEGF and, as a cofactor with IGF and PDGF, has been observed to stimulate angiogenesis.[58,66] TGF-β also inhibits metalloproteinases (MMP-1,-3, and -9) and stimulates tissue inhibitor of metalloproteinase synthesis, which inhibits collagen breakdown.[64,65,71]

TGF-β receptors are particularly enriched in bone and cartilage.[72–76] Immunostaining for TGF-β is most intense during cartilage cell proliferation and endochondral ossification.[74–76] TGF-β modulates bone matrix synthesis by stimulating proliferation of osteoblast precursor cells and bone collagen synthesis.[19] TGF-β induces apoptosis of osteoclasts, thus decreasing bone resorption.[77] Previous studies into the efficacy of in vivo application of TGF-β have shown varying results, and therefore interpretation is difficult because different isoforms, carriers, animal models, and doses of growth factor have been used.[78–82] The bone forming properties of TGF-β seem to be maximized when used with appropriate surgical management (eg, rigid fixation) or combined with a carrier, such as demineralized bone matrix.[3,73]

EPIDERMAL GROWTH FACTOR

A significant number of receptors for EGF are found throughout the epidermis, most prominently in the basal layer, and are also found on endothelial cells, fibroblasts, and smooth muscle cells.[58,83–85] EGF is a chemotactic and a potent mitogen for fibroblasts, epithelial, and endothelial cells.[29,86–88] Additionally, EGF has also been reported to stimulate collagenase activity and angiogensis.[58,85]

The application of topical EGF has been observed to increase epithelialization and decrease healing time in skin graft harvest sites and in venous and diabetic ulcerations.[89–91]

INSULIN-LIKE GROWTH FACTOR

Two IGFs have been identified, IGF-1 and IGF-2.[73] Platelets release IGF-1, which has been seen to promote neovascularization through its effect as a potent chemotactic agent for osteoblasts, vascular smooth muscle, and endothelial cells.[92–94] IGF-1 has also been reported to have a mitogenic effect on fibroblasts, osteocytes, and chondrocytes.[95,96] Furthermore, as a cofactor with PDGF, IGF-1 has been shown to enhance epidermal and dermal growth.[95]

IGF-1 has been reported to play an essential role in bone formation and maintenance.[97,98] IGF-1 has been repeatedly observed to stimulate osteoblast precursors and early osteoblasts, and enhance bone matrix formation from fully differentiated osteoblasts.[99–102] Additionally, IGF-1 promotes type I collagen and matrix protein formation in bone cultures independent of their mitogenic activity.[99] It inhibits collagenase expression by osteoblasts.[99]

IGF-1 and its receptors are widely prevalent in periosteal cells, mesenchymal cells, proliferating chondrocytes, and osteoblasts within fracture callus.[103–106] In animal model studies, the local application of IGF-1, with or without TGF-β1, has been shown to enhance fracture healing.[107–111]

VASCULAR ENDOTHELIAL GROWTH FACTOR

In acute wounds, platelets secrete VEGF-A, which binds VEGF receptor-1 and -2 localized on the endothelial surface of blood vessels.[112–116] VEGF-A is essential in promoting the early steps in angiogenesis, including endothelial chemotaxis and proliferation.[117–121] VEFG-A also stimulates lymphangiogensis.[122]

In cases involving ischemic diabetic limbs, several animal studies involving the administration of VEGF-A have shown a restoration of impaired angiogenesis.[123–127] Additionally, in vivo studies have reported an improvement in reepithelialization of diabetic wounds secondary to enhanced vessel formation with administration of VEGF-A.[128]

Baumgartner and colleagues[129] reported an increase in collateral vessel development in patients who had critical limb ischemia after the intramuscular gene transfer of VEGF-165. However, exogenous application of VEGF-A has been observed to increase vascular leakage and promote disordered and abundant lymphatic formation, suggesting that more research is needed to clarify the efficacy of VEGF-A in wound healing.[130,131]

Although not specifically addressed within the literature regarding PRP and osseous healing, the importance of VEGF in the process of endochondral ossification during osseous maturation has also been documented.[17,132]

AUTOLOGOUS PLATELET-RICH PLASMA

The literature shows that the milieu of growth factors secreted from the α-granules of activated platelets after injury, specifically PDGF, TGF-β, EGF, VEGF-A, and IGF-1, play a critical role in the initiation and process of bone and soft tissue healing. The notion that PRP could provide an autologous source of these essential growth factors and directly benefit bone and soft tissue healing began in the 1990s, largely in the field of oral, periodontal, and spinal surgery.[133–136]

PRP is defined as a sequestration and concentration of platelets within the plasma fraction of autologous blood.[137] Several synonyms for PRP are used in the literature, including platelet-rich concentrate, platelet gel, and platelet releasate.[136,138,139] Although more universal agreement in nomenclature is needed for this platelet derivative, PRP shall be used throughout this article.

Deriving PRP from autologous blood involves several important factors, including platelet concentration ratio, processing technique, quantification of secretory protein concentration, handling, application, and clinical use.[140] The cost of obtaining PRP is also an issue, especially for third-party payers and no definitive current procedure technology (CPT) code exists for this time-consuming and advanced tissue processing technique.

PLATELET CONCENTRATION RATIO

PRP can be considered a substance that supplies more platelets to a wound or injury than what would be produced through a normal physiologic response.[140] In addition to an excess of platelets, PRP also has a full complement of clotting factors, although within normal physiologic limits.[140] Previous reports have stipulated that PRP should achieve a three- to fivefold increase in platelet concentration over baseline, and a PRP count of 1,000,000/µL, as measured in a standard 6-mL aliquot, is regarded as the benchmark for PRP.[11,137,141] Although a three- to fivefold increase over baseline is desirable, several studies have reported concentration ratios of less than 2- and more than 8.5-fold.[12,14,136,137,141]

Experts suggest that platelet counts and growth factor content within PRP do not necessarily follow a linear relationship.[14] Growth factor content is likely to depend on the technique used, the type and extent of injury, the donor's medical and biologic condition (ie, a high variability in individual cellular production), and the storage of growth factors within platelets.[14] Weibrich and colleagues[14] suggest that different individuals may need different platelet concentrations to achieve a comparable biologic effect and concluded that the ability to assess growth factor concentration within PRP is desirable. Furthermore, Eppley[140] reports that a specific desirable platelet concentration recommendation is inherently difficult to establish because of the number of variables and their potential for interactions.

Opponents of PRP cite the potential for wide biologic variation as a reason not to use PRP, specifically in the overexposure of cells to PRP, facilitating a high yield of cells with inadequate differentiation to appropriate cell lines.[142] The fact that most systems do not allow for sterile harvest but instead use aseptic technique must also be considered, because the potential for disease transmission remains.

COLLECTION AND PROCESSING TECHNIQUE

Experts recommend that whole blood collection begin before surgery, because the surgical injury will lead to platelet activation, thus reducing the systemic platelet concentration. Also, the potential to dilute the patient's blood with intravenous fluids is less.[143,144] Given that standard laboratory centrifugation to produce PRP is labor-intensive, maintaining sterility is difficult, and standard cell separators and salvage devices require a unit of autologous blood, more compact systems have been developed to allow easier production and application at the point of care.[133,137,141,143–145] Many surgical procedures only require a modest volume of PRP and these systems produce approximately 6 mL of PRP from 45 to 60 mL of whole blood.[143,146,147]

PRP can be procured from autologous blood through either centrifugation or filtration.[3] Traditionally, centrifugation has formed the basis for PRP production.[140] With centrifugation, anticoagulated autologous whole blood is centrifuged, which separates out the packed red blood cells from the plasma.[148] An additional centrifugation is performed to further separate the PRP from the portion essentially devoid of platelets, termed *platelet-poor plasma* (PPP).[148] PPP can be used clinically as a fibrin sealant for hemostasis.[143,144] Although centrifugation has traditionally been the standard for obtaining the PRP fraction, caution is needed because of the potential for platelet fragmentation and premature activation during the spinning process, resulting in compromised bioactivity.[12,141]

Various optimal spin cycles have been advocated for this process. Landesberg and colleagues[149] determined optimal platelet enrichment with first and second spin cycles of 200 g for 10 minutes, as opposed to 250 g, which resulted in a failure to suspend adequate platelet quantities. Efeoglu and colleagues[150] reported a threefold higher platelet count than the Landesberg method for both PRP and PPP, with a first spin of 300 g for 10 minutes and a second spin of 5000 g for 5 minutes.[149,150]

Gonshor[141] recommends using acid citrate dextrose type A (ACD-A) anticoagulant and low gravity forces during centrifugation to maintain the integrity of the platelet membrane. Regarding premature activation, Eppley and colleagues[12] used P-selectin, a platelet surface marker for platelet activation, to show that centrifugation does not result in premature activation of platelets in PRP preparation using this method.

PRP without centrifugation can be performed using a filtration device.[3] Previous filtration devices have been criticized for being too vigorous or using pediatric dialysis filters and cell saver, leading to problems with fragmentation and early activation of platelets.[137] Newer filtration devices use a cell-sensitive filtration system and are comparatively atraumatic.[3] Approximately 60 mL of autologous whole blood is mixed with an anticoagulant, such as ACD-A, and this combination is then passed through a compact filter system and then backflushed, yielding approximately 6 to 7 mL of PRP. This method of acquiring PRP is reported to be 40% faster than centrifugation and yield equivalent concentrations of platelets.[3] However, more comparative studies are required before a definitive recommendation of centrifugation or filtration can be made. Roukis and colleagues[151] provides a comprehensive review of available PRP systems.

PLATELET-RICH PLASMA QUANTIFICATION

The potential efficacy of PRP is dependent on the level of growth factors secreted from activated platelets.[12,14] The level of growth factors released depends on the actual concentration of these factors within the α granules, the processing technique, and the proportion or completeness of activated platelets.[12,152,153] When compared with baseline values, a three- to fourfold increase in growth factor levels is reported in PRP.[12,14,154] A correlation does not seen to exist between individual growth factor levels and age or gender.[14]

The relationship between growth factor and platelet concentration levels has been investigated, with varying results, but a general linear trend exists between increasing levels of growth factors and increasing levels of platelets.[12,14] However, Eppley and colleagues[12] and Weibrich and colleagues[14] caution against relying on using platelet concentration to predict resultant growth factor levels because of the variability of different systems and the variability inherent in platelet activation and binding of growth factors to the terminal clot.[3,140]

APPLICATION OF PLATELET-RICH PLASMA

Once the PRP is produced, it is stable for approximately 8 hours in the anticoagulated state.[11,155] For the platelets within the plasma fraction to become activated and degranulate, and thus release their growth factors, an exogenous application of 1000 IU of bovine thrombin per milliliter solution of 10% calcium chloride must be added.[12,136,143] After this, the clot that forms provides the vehicle that contains the growth factor milieu for delivery to the area of injury or site of therapy.[140]

Depending on the system used, the process of activation can be performed by adding the thrombin or calcium chloride to the syringe containing the PRP, followed by agitation of the syringe and then application to the site of therapy.[136] Alternatively, a dual syringe mixing system can be used, in which the plungers of a 10-mL syringe housing the PRP and a separate 1-mL syringe containing the activating solution are depressed together, thereby mixing both solutions as they exit and are applied to the site of therapy.[143]

Although not an issue with the dual syringe mechanism, the activated PRP is recommended to be used within 10 minutes of clot initiation given the fact that platelets release the contents of the α granules shortly after activation.[11]

The production of antibodies to clotting factors V, XI, and thrombin have been reported after exposure to bovine product to provide hemostasis to open, bleeding vessels.[156–158] However, no published evidence exists that of cross-reaction in the application of PRP, probably because of the elimination of bovine factor Va from the processing of bovine thrombin and that its use in PRP prevents its exposure to the systemic circulation.[140,159]

CLINICAL USE
Platelet-rich Plasma in Bone and Bone Graft Healing

In vitro studies
Arpornmaeklong and colleagues[160] seeded porous collagen carriers with marrow-derived bone-forming cells from rats and exposed these to different concentrations of PRP, PPP, and bone morphogenic protein (BMP). Although those collagen carriers with PRP show a dose-dependent cell proliferation, an overall inhibition of osteogenic differentiation of marrow-derived preosteoblasts was seen, showing that PRP is not a substitute for BMP-2 osteogenic induction.[160] Additionally, Slapnicka and colleagues[161] did not show significant increases in proliferation of human osteoblasts treated with activated and nonactivated PRP compared with controls. However, activated PRP resulted in higher proliferation of osteoblasts than nonactivated PRP.[161]

In a study of the effect of PRP on stromal stem cell (SCC) proliferation and differentiation, Lucarelli and colleagues[162] observed that 10% PRP is sufficient to induce logarithmic SSC growth compared with controls. After proliferation, they were also able to show a threefold increase in the number of alkaline phosphatase–positive cells and induced mineralization, consistent with differentiation of osteochondroprogenitor cells.[162]

Kanno and colleagues[163] also showed favorable effects of PRP on human osteoblast-like cells in a dose-dependent manner, with enhanced levels of procollagen type I, osteopontin, osteoprotegerin, and core-binding factor α 1 mRNA, a critical regulator of osteoblast differentiation. Alkaline phosphatase activity, although initially suppressed during the cell growth, was strongly enhanced when the cells reached confluence.[163]

More recently, Tomoyasu and colleagues[164] showed that PRP stimulated osteoblast differentiation of myoblasts and osteoblastic cells in the presence of BMP-2, -4, and -6 or -7 in three-dimensional cultures using hydroxyapatite or collagen scaffolds, indicating that platelets contain growth factors for proliferation and potentiators for BMP-dependent osteoblastic differentiation.[164]

Animal studies
Similar to in vitro studies, the results of animal studies are divided with regard to the efficacy of PRP. In two recent studies in immuno-compromised nude mice, Ranly and colleagues[165,166] observed a reduction in osteoinductivity of demineralized bone matrix impregnated with PRP implanted within muscle. PRP was observed to decrease osteoinductivity of demineralized bone matrix with high osteoinductive activity and had no effect on bone matrix with low inductivity.[166]

Gandhi and colleagues[142] examined growth factor expression in the fracture callus and the effect of percutaneously injected PRP on fracture healing in Wistar rats that spontaneously develop insulin-dependent diabetes mellitus. They saw a significant reduction in PDGF, TGF-β1, IGF-I, and VEGF in diabetic fracture callus compared with nondiabetic fracture callus. Injection of PRP was shown to normalize early diabetic fracture callus and improved the late parameters of diabetic fracture healing. PRP-treated diabetic rats exhibited bone formation that was histologically similar to nondiabetic rats.[142]

Weibrich and colleagues[153] evaluated the effect of platelet concentrations of PRP on bone regeneration after insertion of a titanium screw in the femur of white rabbits versus controls. They showed that concentrations of approximately 1,000,000/μL are required to achieve advantageous biologic effects; however, a suboptimal effect was seen at lower concentrations and an inhibitory effect at higher concentrations. Overall, no differences were seen in the bone/implant contact rates between the test and the control side.[153]

In a study evaluating the effect of PRP on autogenous bone graft remodeling during sinus augmentation in a rabbit model, Butterfield and colleagues[167] failed to show a direct stimulatory effect on healing.

Several studies have shown a positive effect of PRP in the healing of critical-size defects and bone grafts in a rabbit model. Kim and colleagues[168] showed increased bone formation when PRP was applied to bovine bone graft for calvarial defects. Kasten and colleagues[169] investigated bone healing in critical-sized diaphyseal radius defects and showed that allogenic PRP improves bone healing with calcium-deficient hydroxyapatite with and without the addition of mesenchymal stem cells. Kroese-Deutman and colleagues[170] observed a stimulatory benefit of PRP when used with autologous bone chips and titanium fiber mesh in a rabbit radial defect model.

Also in a rabbit model, Aghaloo and colleagues[171–173] reported a trend toward increased bone density in cranial defects at 1, 2, and 4 months when PRP was applied with freeze-dried mineralized and demineralized bone graft,[171] xenograft,[172] and auotgraft[173]; however, these findings were not statistically significant.

In a domestic pig model, Thorwarth and colleagues[174] used immunohistochemistry to show increased osteocalcin, osteopontin, and BMP-2 production in defined defects filled with collagen lyophilisat and PRP versus autogenous bone. However, several studies involving osseous defects, sinus augmentation, and dental implants in pigs have shown no benefit with the application of PRP in combination with various graft or filler materials.[175–178]

Fennis and colleagues[159] showed considerable enhancement in bone healing in the goat model after applying PRP to autogenous graft in mandibular defects fixated with osteosynthesis plates. However, Mooren and colleagues[179] showed through histologic and histomorphometric examination that early and late bone healing in critical defects in the foreheads of goats were not enhanced with PRP and autogenous graft bone versus graft alone.

Several studies involving dog and sheep models have also questioned the effectiveness of PRP in osseous healing.[180–183] In two separate studies, Jensen and colleagues[180,181] found no significant effect of PRP alone[180] or when mixed with bone allograft[180,181] on implant fixation or bone formation in a dog model. Also in a canine model, Choi and colleagues[182] evaluated the effect of PRP on autogenous bone graft regeneration after bilateral mandibular premolar teeth extraction. They found that adding PRP to autogenous bone graft within the defects delayed bone formation compared with the contralateral control side.

Sarkar and colleagues[183] reported on the effect of PRP on bone regeneration in a critical diaphyseal long-bone defect in a sheep model, supplied with PRP and collagen carrier versus collagen carrier alone. Bone volume, mineral density, mechanical rigidity, and histology of the newly formed bone in the defect did not differ significantly between the PRP-treated and the control groups, and no effect of PRP on bone formation was observed.[183]

Human studies: oral maxillofacial surgery

In human subjects, most literature on PRP is in the field of oral and maxillofacial surgery. In a randomized controlled trial, Marx and colleagues[136] were able to show radiographic maturation rates 1.62 to 2.16 times faster in mandibular defects treated with cancellous cellular marrow graft with PRP versus marrow grafts alone. Robiony and colleagues,[184] also showed the effectiveness of PRP in mandibular reconstruction in a case series of five subjects undergoing distraction osteogenesis for severe atrophy of the edentulous mandible. After PRP and autogenous iliac crest graft interposition into the distraction defect, planned distraction height was attained. The authors concluded that a significant enhancement in osseous regeneration occurred.[184]

The literature dealing with PRP in maxillary sinus augmentation is divided. In one case series and one randomized trial, Kassolis and colleagues[185,186] reported on the enhancement of sinus augmentation with the application of PRP and freeze-dried bone graft. The enhancement of bone regeneration was also shown in several other case series involving PRP in sinus augmentation with allogenic or autogenous graft.[187–189] In a case-control series, Thor and colleagues[190] observed significantly more bone formation in the PRP and autogenous bone–grafted site than the contralateral control side using histologic investigation at 3 months. The benefit was not observed at 6 months, suggesting that the value of PRP is in the early phase of bone healing.[191] However, two recent studies by Schaaf and colleagues[192,193] have shown no positive effect of PRP on bone grafting in sinus floor augmentation. In a prospective, randomized controlled trial, Schaaf and colleagues[192] reported no difference in bone density using CT, panoramic radiography, and histomorphometry at 4 months postintervention versus controls.

Human studies: orthopaedic surgery

Kitoh and colleagues[194–196] have investigated the potential for PRP in combination with bone marrow cells (BMC) in distraction osteogenesis of the femur and/or tibia, for subjects with achondroplasia, hypochondroplasia or congenital pseudarthrosis. In their retrospective comparative studies, transplantation of the PRP and BMC's was performed at the lengthening and consolidation period in each subject. The authors concluded that transplantation of PRP and BMC's resulted in acceleration of new bone regeneration during distraction osteogenesis, decreased treatment times and reduced complications[194,195]

PRP has also been employed in spinal fusions.[134,197–199] In their retrospective case series, Lowery and colleagues[134] applied PRP with autograft and coralline hydroxyapatite to all posterior lumbar fusions, and with autograft, coralline hydroxyapatite, and intradiscal spacers for intradiscal fusions. What methods were used for evaluation is unclear, although the authors conclude that PRP promotes early maturation of osseous fusion when used as an adjunct with autograft.[134]

In a prospective series, Jenis and colleagues[199] compared PRP with allogenic graft versus traditional autogenous graft for lumbar interbody fusion using clinical and radiologic parameters as outcome measures at 12 and 24 months. They reported no significant difference between treatment groups and concluded that allogenic graft with PRP is a viable alternative to autogenous graft harves.[199] Carreon and colleagues[198] also failed to show an enhancement in lumbar fusion using autogenous bone graft with or without PRP. In a single-blind, retrospective radiographic review of autogenous bone graft with or without PRP in lumbar fusion, Weiner and colleagues[200] observed a decreased fusion rate when PRP was added to the autogenous graft.

The use of PRP has also been used to treat nonunions.[201] In a prospective case series with historical controls, Mariconda and colleagues[201] injected PRP into the nonunion site of 20 patients who had tibial, humeral, or forearm atrophic nonunions treated with percutaneous stabilization with unilateral external fixators. The authors failed to show a difference in the mean time to radiographic consolidation between historical controls and subjects receiving percutaneous injection of PRP.[201]

Human studies: foot and ankle surgery

Gandhi and colleagues[148] were among the first to use PRP in subjects diagnosed with a nonunion of a fracture of the foot and ankle that was present for a minimum of 4 months. They applied PRP with autogenous bone graft to the sites of nonunion followed by standard osteosynthesis techniques. The authors observed a resolution of nonunion at a mean of 60 days.

These authors also compared growth factor levels at the site of the nonunion with those from a cohort of fresh fractures. A significant reduction of growth factors at the nonunion site was observed compared with those present at the hematoma at the site of the fresh fracture.[148] The authors suggest that the addition of PRP to the nonunion site brings critical growth factors to the region, resulting in the positive influence of nonunion resolution.[148]

Coetzee and colleagues[202] reported on the benefit of PRP in the syndesmosis union rate in total ankle arthroplasty. In their retrospective comparative series, the authors compared the syndesmosis union rate between 66 subjects who received PRP-augmented autogenous grafts and 114 nonaugmented historical controls. CT and plain radiography was the primary outcome measure. The historical controls had a 61% and 85% fusion rate at 8 weeks and 6 months, respectively, with a resultant 15% rate of nonunion. In contrast, the syndesmotic fusion rate in subjects receiving PRP augmented autogenous bone grafts showed a 76% union rate at 8 weeks and a 97% union rate at 6 months, resulting in a 3% nonunion rate. A statistically significant difference in the time to union and a reduction in delayed and non unions was observed favoring PRP-augmented syndesmosis fusion. In addition to this, Coetzee and colleagues[202] observed a higher syndesmosis fusion rate in the subset of tobacco smokers within the PRP-augmented treatment group (80%) compared with the subset of smokers within the historical controls (50%) at 6 months.

Barrow and Pomeroy[203] also reported on a prospective case series of 20 subjects who received PRP to enhance syndesmosis fusion in total ankle arthroplasty. The authors reported an 85% union rate at 8 weeks and a 100% union rate at 6 months postoperation, based on radiographic evidence of union.

Bibbo and colleagues[204] reported on union rates in their study evaluating the use of PRP in high-risk elective foot and ankle surgery. The study included 62 patients (123 procedures) who had at least one identifiable risk factor for poor bone healing. Risk factors included diabetes with neuropathy, tobacco smoking, immunosuppression, malnutrition, alcohol abuse, osteomyelitis, history of impaired osseous healing, multiple same site surgeries, or high-energy trauma. PRP was applied to each fusion site, with 56 procedures requiring a form of autogenous or allogenic graft. Of their cohort, 58 subjects (94%) or 116 fusion sites (94%) underwent successful fusion with a mean time to union of 41 days. No significant difference was seen between bone grafted and non–bone grafted fusion sites. Additionally, no significant difference was seen in fusion rates between anatomic regions (ankle 95%, rearfoot 92%, midfoot 94%, and forefoot 94%). The investigators concluded that the use of PRP in high-risk patients undergoing foot and ankle surgery may help achieve an acceptable time to union.

In a retrospective study, Grant and colleagues[205] compared the fusion rates of Charcot's foot reconstruction surgeries in 50 cases in which the Interpore Cross AGF system (Interpore Cross, Irvine, California) or the Symphony PRP concentration system (DePuy, Warsaw, Indiana) was used. Charcot's foot reconstruction cases included 14 ankle/tibiocalcaneal fusion, 14 triple arthrodeses, 12 midtarsal arthrodeses, and 10 Lisfranc arthrodeses. A combination of allogenic and autogenous bone graft, internal large-diameter screw fixation, external fixation, and PRP was used. Grant and colleagues[205] reported that overall incidence of solid fusion of the operative sites was 43% for the ankle/tibiocalcaneal fusions, 85% for triple arthrodesis, 72% for the midtarsal fusions, and 83% for the Lisfranc's joint. Stratification of devices showed an 83% fusion rate with the use of Interpore Cross AGF and a 62% fusion rate with Symphony.[206]

PLATELET-RICH PLASMA AND WOUND HEALING

The process of wound healing is manifold and comprises a series of complex interactions and events, not fully understood, though well orchestrated through signaling proteins.[7] Historically, wound healing has been divided into three broad phases, including hemostasis and inflammation, proliferation, and maturation.[7] During the initial inflammatory phase, collagen exposed after wound formation results in a blood clot composed of collagen, platelets, thrombin, and fibronectin. This process provides hemostasis and a reservoir to release and concentrate cytokines and growth factors, which in turn coordinates cellular chemotaxis, proliferation, angiogenesis, provisional matrix formation, epithelialization, and maturation.[7] Platelet activation, cytokine and growth factor release, and subsequent chemotaxis and cellular differentiation are critical to effect normal wound healing. PRP, which is exceedingly rich in growth factors, would seem to be ideally suited for augmenting wound healing.

In Vitro Studies

Kakudo and colleagues[207] examined the potential of PRP on human adipose-derived stem cells and human dermal fibroblasts. Activated and nonactivated PRP and PPP were prepared and applied to cultures of human adipose-derived stem cells and human dermal fibroblasts and cultured for 7 days. The application of activated PRP and PPP resulted in significant proliferation of both cell types compared with their nonactivated forms, with activated PRP having the strongest proliferative effect. Kakudo and colleagues[207] observed a dose-dependent relationship with the effect of PRP on proliferation, with 1% to 5% having a maximal effect and a decreasing effect observed with higher concentrations of 10% to 20%.

Graziani and colleagues[208] evaluated the effect of different concentrations of PRP on human oral osteoblast and fibroblast function in vitro. Primary human cultures of the respective cell types were exposed to both activated and nonactivated PRP, including various concentrations of PRP, and PRP-stimulated cell proliferation was observed in both osteoblasts and fibroblasts.

Similar to Kakudo and colleagues,[207] Graziani and colleagues[208] showed a dose-dependent maximum effect with a PRP concentration of 2.5 above baseline, with higher concentrations resulting in a reduction of cell proliferation. Increased concentrations resulted in reduced proliferation and a suboptimal effect on osteoblast function. The investigators concluded that different PRP concentrations may impact the results that can be obtained in vivo.[208]

Lundquist and colleagues[209] examined the effects of platelet-rich fibrin (PRF) on cultured normal human dermal fibroblasts. PRF contains a platelet-rich concentrate with fibrin(ogen), and experts have postulated that the addition of fibrin and fibrinogen may reduce the susceptibility of endogenous polypeptidic growth factors to proteolytic degradation.[209] The effects of PRF were compared with supernatant from thrombin-activated platelet concentrate, recombinant human platelet-derived growth factor (rhPDGF) isoforms, and a homologous fibrin sealant in cultured normal human dermal fibroblasts.

Lundquist and colleagues[209] showed that PRF strongly stimulated the synthesis of type I collagen in dermal fibroblasts and that at least two growth factors are protected from proteolytic degradation in PRFs. The investigators concluded that this may be advantageous in the treatment of chronic wounds characterized by high proteinase activity.[209]

Animal Studies

Several animal studies investigated the effect of PRP on wound healing. Phillips and colleagues[210] observed increased leukocyte margination and angiogenesis in sponges soaked with platelet-derived wound-healing factors and implanted into rats. In another rodent model, Tanaka and colleagues[211] investigated a novel wound dressing consisting of concentrated plasma proteins and platelet releasate applied to excisional skin wounds in genetically healing-impaired mice. They observed that wounds treated with concentrated plasma proteins and platelet releasate decreased significantly at 10 days compared with controls (65% versus 94% of original size, respectively), including an increased vascular density.[212] Additionally, Moulin and colleagues[213] also showed the effectiveness of PRP on cutaneous wound healing in diabetic rats. Histologically, they observed improvement in tissue repair and a restoration of the impaired healing steps in the treated diabetic rat skin compared with the untreated skin.[213]

Vermeulen and colleages[214] presented the use of PRP and autologous keratinocytes on 20 full-thickness wounds in a pig model. They observed a significantly enhanced reepithelialization of wounds in the group treated with PRP and keratinocytes, compared with the PRP-only and control groups. However, immunofluorescence microscopy showed more granulation tissue in the group treated with PRP and keratinocytes than in controls, suggesting PRP enhances deposition of matrix molecules in the inflammatory and proliferative phase of wound healing, and the combination of PRP and autologous keratinocytes can enhance reepithelialization and revascularization.[214]

Carter and colleagues[215] investigated the potential of platelet-derived factors to enhance wound healing in full-thickness cutaneous wounds created below the knee and hock of a thoroughbred horse. In this case-control study, wounds were treated with PRP gel or left untreated, and both were dressed with a sterile nonadherent gauze and circumferential bandage. Sequential wound biopsies were collected at days 7, 36, and 79 postwounding. PRP gel-treated wounds at day 7 expressed intense cytokeratin-10 staining compared with the control wound, and at day 79, the PRP wounds contained abundant, dense, collagen bundles oriented parallel to each other and to the overlying epithelium. Control tissues contained fewer collagen fibers and were oriented randomly.[215]

In a rabbit model investigation, Chandra and colleagues[216] applied PRP to one of a pair of skin flaps dissected on the backs of 12 rabbits. Punch biopsy specimens were obtained at 1-, 2-, and 3-week intervals. An overall increase in inflammation was seen in PRP wounds, with significant increases in subdermal eosinophilia; however, no significant differences were noted regarding degree of fibrosis or collagen deposition between wounds.[216]

Human Studies

Man and colleagues[143] showed that PPP and PRP used in cosmetic facial flap surgery in 20 patients resulted in a decreased need for drains, reduction of postoperative swelling and erythema, and accelerated primary flap healing. Powell and colleagues[217] implemented PRP in a prospective case-control series of eight participants undergoing deep-plane rhytidectomy. Staged postoperative photographs were analyzed in a blinded fashion by three plastic surgeons. Although not statistically significant, the results showed less edema and ecchymosis in the PRP-treated side, particularly in the early phases of healing.[217]

Marx[11] reported on the application of PRP with standard treatment for two side-by-side, split-thickness skin graft harvest sites (0.016 inch) from a single patient's thigh. At 6 days postprocedure, the harvest site treated with PRP displayed significantly less peripheral edema than the control site. Furthermore, a thin epithelial covering was evident at the PRP site compared with a less than 5% covering of the control site. The control site showed no evidence of epithelial budding with immature fibroblasts and macrophages. The PRP-treated site showed mature epithelial budding and a mature dermis. Differences were also evident at 6 months, with increased scarring and a greater loss of pigmented cells at the control graft harvest site.[11]

In a randomized trial investigating the effect of PRP on epithelialization of donor sites and meshed split-thickness skin autografts for 20 leg ulcers, Danielsen and colleagues[218] observed no statistically significant differences in macroscopic epithelialization between PRP and control dressing for graft harvest wounds or skin autografts, including bacterial flora count and patient-reported pain.

Hom and colleagues[219] evaluated the healing of acute full-thickness punch wounds treated with PRP versus conventional therapy in 80 wounds occurring on the thighs of healthy volunteers. In this prospective, single-blind, case-control study, PRP was applied topically to one thigh (five biopsy sites) and an antibiotic ointment or semiocclusive dressing was applied on the other thigh (five sites). Over a 42-day period, the PRP-treated sites had statistically increased wound closure compared with controls; however, over time cellularity, cellular replication, granulation tissue, vascularity, and epithelialization was observed to be similar to controls.[219]

Kazakos and colleagues[220] assessed the benefits of using PRP to treat acute soft tissue wounds in traumatized limbs, including open fractures, closed fractures with skin necrosis, and friction burns. This study randomized 59 patients who had acute wounds to receive conventional dressings or the application of PRP. Clinical end points were the healing rate or time required for adequate tissue regeneration to undergo reconstructive plastic surgery. Through weeks 1 to 3, the wound healing rate was significantly faster for the PRP-treated group, and the mean time to plastic reconstruction in the PRP group was 21.3 days compared with 40.6 days for the control group. The authors concluded that PRP can be a valuable aid for treating acute trauma wounds.[220]

Several studies report favorable results in chronic wounds treated with PRP, including a favorable effect on limb salvage rates among high-risk patients.[221–224]

In the first clinical demonstration of PDGFs to promote wound healing, Knighton and colleagues[225] evaluated the effects of PRP on 95 chronic wounds in 49 patients, present for a mean of 198 weeks. After application of PRP, 100% healing was achieved in all patients within 10.6 weeks.[225] Another study by Knighton and colleagues[226] was conducted with 32 participants who had chronic, nonhealing cutaneous wounds of the lower extremity. In this prospective, single-blind trial, the authors randomized participants to a PRP or placebo intervention for 8 weeks, with epithelialization as the end point. Epithelialization was observed in 81% of participants treated with PRP, compared with 15% in controls at 8 weeks. After this point, the control group crossed over to PRP treatment, and all patients subsequently achieved epithelialization at a mean of 7.1 weeks. The authors observed a statistically significant effect of topically applied PRP on the repair of chronic, nonhealing, cutaneous ulcers.[226]

Other investigators have reported clinical success with the use of PRP in recalcitrant ulcers. Atri and colleagues[227] reported on the use of PRP in 23 participants with 27 diabetic or venous stasis ulcerations present for a mean period of 25 weeks. After 3 months of controlled wound care consisting of saline and silver sulfadiazine applications, only 3 ulcerations healed, leaving 24 persistent ulcerations that failed to achieve 50% epithelialization. These residual ulcerations were subsequently treated with PRP and silver sulfadiazine, and achieved complete healing at a mean of 9.7 weeks. Those who had diabetes-related ulceration healed faster (mean, 6.9 weeks) than the venous stasis ulcerations (mean, 14.0 weeks).[227]

Steed and colleagues[228] assessed the efficacy of PRP on diabetic neuropathic foot ulcers present for greater than 8 weeks in 13 participants randomized to receive homologous PRP or placebo consisting of normal saline gauze applications. Wounds were excised before intervention and the time to complete epithelialization was achieved by week 15 in five of seven participants receiving PRP, as opposed to one in six treated with placebo by week 20. Additionally, by week 20, an average reduction in ulcer volume by 94% was seen versus 73% for PRP and placebo treatment groups, respectively.[228]

Driver and colleagues[229] evaluated the safety and efficacy of PRP for the treatment of nonhealing diabetic foot ulcers in a multicenter, double-blind, prospective, randomized controlled trial. This study randomized 40 participants who had a foot ulcer for longer than 4 weeks to receive PRP or saline placebo dressing twice weekly for 12 weeks or until complete healing occurred. Wounds were considered healed at 1 week after wound closure. Of the 40 participants (40 wounds), significantly more wounds treated with PRP experienced wound closure (81.3%) compared with the control group (42.1%). The authors concluded that when good standards of care are used, nonhealing diabetic foot ulcers treated with PRP can be expected to heal.[229]

In another double-blind, placebo-controlled, multicenter study, Holloway and colleagues[230] randomized 70 participants (70 wounds) to receive either placebo or diluted homologous PRP of 1:10, 1:30, or 1:100 concentration. Of wounds treated with PRP, 63% achieved closure as opposed to 29% receiving placebo intervention. The authors observed that the group receiving the 1:100-diluted PRP showed the most efficacious healing, with an 80% healing rate.

In contrast, a report by Krupski and colleagues[231] concluded that treatment of chronic wounds with autologous platelet-derived wound healing factors (PDWHF) provides no additional benefit over traditional therapy. This prospective, double-blind study, randomized 18 patients who had 26 lower extremity wounds refractory to conventional therapy to receive topical PDWHF or placebo. Participants were afflicted with diabetes (78%), peripheral arterial disease (72%), or venous disease (28%). The investigators reported spuriously high ankle brachial indices of 0.93 for placebo and 1.03 for the intervention group. Wounds were present for a minimum of 8 weeks and initially underwent extensive debridement before intervention. The wounds were measured and photographed at weekly intervals. The investigators also observed a poor healing rate of 33% for controls and 24% for wounds treated with autologous PDWHF, and concluded that this preparation provides no additional benefit for healing chronic wounds.

PLATELET-RICH PLASMA IN CARTILAGE REPAIR

Few in vitro studies have investigated the effect of PRP on cartilage metabolism and proliferation. In a study aimed at determining the plausibility of using PRP material for engineering cartilage, Akeda and colleagues[232] examined the effects of 10% PRP, 10% PPP, or 10% fetal bone serum on cell proliferation and matrix synthesis by porcine chondrocytes. The investigators observed a small but significant increase in DNA content, which is a marker of cell proliferation, and a marked increase in proteoglycan and collagen synthesis in the PRP-treated chondrocytes. These findings indicate that PRP has potential as an anabolic source for stimulating chondrocytes in engineered cartilage tissue.[232] Other investigators have observed increased chondrocyte proliferation with platelet lysate in vitro.[233–235]

Saito and colleagues[236] showed that intraarticular injections of PRP in gelatin hydrogel microspheres significantly suppressed progression of osteoarthritis in a rabbit knee model morphologically and histologically. Nakagawa and colleagues[237] observed a significant increase in type II collagen synthesis in chondrocytes harvested from human knee arthroplasty specimens, suggesting the usefulness of PRP in treating cartilage defects.

PLATELET-RICH PLASMA IN TENDON REPAIR

In an in vitro study investigating the effect of dose-dependent PRP application to cultured human tenocytes, de Mos and colleagues[238] showed that the application of both PRP and PPP increased cell number and total collagen production, with PRP up-regulating matrix metalloproteinases-1 and -3. The investigators suggest that in vivo, PRP might accelerate tenocyte catabolic demarcation of traumatically injured tendon matrices and promote angiogenesis and fibrovascular callus.[238] Other investigators have shown increased tendon cell proliferation in vitro.[239]

Several studies have shown the efficacy of PRP in repair of the Achilles tendon in a rat model.[240–242] In a surgically induced Achilles tendon defect, PRP was observed to increase tendon callus strength and stiffness by 30% at 1 week postintervention.[240] In another rat model,[242] transected Achilles tendons treated with PRP showed a 42% increase in force to failure, 90% increase in energy, and 61% increase in ultimate stress compared with saline after 14 days postintervention.

Mishra and Pavelko[243] reported a significant improvement in participants experiencing elbow epicondylar tendinosis after a single injection of PRP versus bupivacaine plain. At 8 weeks, 6 months, and mean final follow-up of 25 months, participants receiving PRP had a significantly greater reduction in pain compared with those receiving bupivacaine, measured using the visual analog pain scale.[243]

DISCUSSION

Growth factors released from the α granules of activated platelets are integral in the coordination and regulation of multiple cell types in bone and soft tissue healing. The therapeutic application of supraphysiologic levels of platelets, and ultimately their contents, to bone and soft tissue injury has gained interest in the recent 2 decades. The benefits of PRP include its ease of production at the point of care; comparable cost-effectiveness compared with other orthobiologics for osseous augmentation, such as bone growth stimulators and rhBMP; and its low reported morbidity and associated complications.[148]

A significant literature dedicated to the evaluation of PRP undoubtedly shows its beneficial effects on the microscopic and therapeutic events in bone and wound healing. More recent investigations into cartilage and tendon healing are promising. Unfortunately, the literature contains little consistency regarding particular systems used and the procurement, quantity, and therapeutic protocol, making interpretation of the literature for clinical application inherently difficult. Additionally, meaningful conclusions for clinical use in bone and joint surgery are problematic given the diverse success rates among the foot and ankle, the spine, and the maxillofacial literature. Although a volume of studies involve human participants, except for those involving the management of chronic wounds or ulceration, only a relatively small proportion of well-designed studies exist and even fewer for the foot and ankle. More well-designed, prospective, rigorous clinical trials using consistent techniques may lead to more conclusive and therefore clinically generalizable recommendations.

SUMMARY

According to the modest current evidence within the foot and ankle literature, use of PRP has significant potential for treating patients at risk for nonunion, acute traumatic wounds and chronic ulceration refractory to local wound care. Although PRP has shown benefit in the several arenas, good technique with respect to appropriate osteosynthesis or wound care is mandatory.

REFERENCES

1. Behnke O, Forer A. From megakaryocytes to platelets: platelet morphogenesis takes place in the bloodstream. Eur J Haematol Suppl 1998;61(1):3–23.
2. Italiano JE Jr, Hartwig JH. Megakaryocyte and platelet structure. Chapter 105. In: Hoffman R, editor. Hematology: basic principles and practice. 4th Edition. Philadelphia: Elsevier, Churchill-Livingstone; 2005. p. 1872–80.
3. Mehta S, Watson JT. Platelet rich concentrate: basic science and current clinical applications. J Orthop Trauma 2008;22(6):433–8.
4. Pagana KD, Pagana TJ. Blood studies: platelet count. Chapter 2. In: Pagana KD, Pagana TJ, editors. Mosby's Manual of Diagnostic and laboratory Tests. St Louis (IL): Mosby Elsevier; 2006. p. 409–12.
5. Harrison P, Cramer EM. Platelet alpha-granules. Blood Rev 1993;7(1):52–62.
6. Plow EF, Abrams CS. Chapter 106-the molecular basis for platelet function. Chapter 106. In: Hoffman R, editor. Hematology: basic principles and practice. 4th Edition. Philadelphia: Elsevier, Churchill, Livingstone; 2005. p. 1881–98.
7. Broughton G II, Janis JE, Attinger CE. Wound healing: an overview. Plast Reconstr Surg 2006;117(Suppl 7S):1eS–32eS.
8. Broughton G II, Janis JE, Attinger CE. The basic science of wound healing. Plast Reconstr Surg 2006;117(Suppl):12S–34S.
9. Witte M, Barbul A. General principles of wound healing. Surg Clin North Am 1997;77(3):509–28.
10. Diegelman RF, Evans MC. Wound healing: an overview of acute fibrotic and delayed healing. Front Biosci 2004;9:283–9.
11. Marx RE. Platelet-rich plasma: evidence to support its use. J Oral Maxillofac Surg 2004;62(4):489–96.
12. Eppley BL, Woodell JE, Higgins J. Platelet quantification and growth factor analysis from platelet-rich plasma: implications for wound healing. Plast Reconstr Surg 2004;114(11):1502–8.
13. Schmidmaier G, Herrmann S, Green J, et al. Quantitative assessment of growth factors in reaming aspirate, iliac crest, and platelet preparation. Bone 2006;39(5):1156–63.

14. Weibrich G, Kleis WK, Hafner G, et al. Growth factor levels in platelet-rich plasma and correlations with donor age, sex, and platelet count. J Craniomax-illofac Surg 2002;30(2):97–102.
15. Ratnoff OD, Davie EW. Waterfall sequence for intrinsic blood clotting. Science 1964;145:1310–2.
16. Froum SJ, Wallace SS, Tarnow DP, et al. Effect of platelet-rich plasma on bone growth and osseointegration in human maxillary sinus grafts: three bilateral case reports. Int J Periodontics Restorative Dent 2002;22(1):45–53.
17. Bennett SP, Griffiths GD, Schor AM, et al. Growth factors in the treatment of diabetic foot ulcers. Br J Surg 2003;90(2):133–46.
18. Pierce G, Mustoe T, Altrock B, et al. Role of platelet-derived growth factor in wound healing. J Cell Biochem 1991;45(4):319–26.
19. Canalis E, McCarthy TL, Centerlla M. Effects of Platelet-derived growth factor on bone formation in vitro. J Cell Physiol 1989;140(3):530–7.
20. Heldin CH, Westermark B. Mechanism of action and in vivo role of platelet-derived growth factor. Physiol Rev 1999;79(4):1283–316.
21. Heldin CH, Westermark B. PDGF-like growth factors in autocrine simulation of growth. J Cell Physiol 1987;133(Suppl 5):31–4.
22. Lin H, Chen B, Sun W, et al. The effect of collagen-targeting platelet-derived growth factor on cellularization and vascularization of collagen scaffolds. Biomaterials 2006;27(33):5708–14.
23. Acevedo JI. Fixation of metatarsal osteotomies in the treatment of hallux valgus. Foot Ankle Clin 2000;5(3):451–68.
24. Rhee S, Grinnel F. P21-activated kinase 1: convergence point in PDGF- and LPA-stimulated collagen matrix contraction by human fibroblasts. J Cell Biol 2006;172(3):423–32.
25. Uutela M, Wirzenius M, Paavonen K, et al. PDGF-D induces macrophage recruitment, increased interstitial pressure, and blood vessel maturation during angiogenesis. Blood 2004;104(10):3198–204.
26. Jinnin M, Ihn H, Mimura Y, et al. Regulation of fibrogenic/fibrolytic genes by platelet-derived growth factor C, a novel growth factor, in human dermal fibroblasts. J Cell Biol 2005;202(2):510–7.
27. Rabhi-Sabile S, Pidard D, Lawler J, et al. Proteolysis of thrombospondin during cathepsin-G-induced platelet aggregation: functional role of the 165-kDa carboxy-terminal fragment. FEBS Lett 1996;386(1):82–6.
28. Krishnaswami S, Ly QP, Rothman VL, et al. Thrombospondin-1 promotes proliferative healing through stabilization of PDGF. J Surg Res 2002;107(1):124–30.
29. Ando Y, Jensen PJ. Epidermal growth factor and insulin-like growth factor I enhance keratinocyte migration. J Invest Dermatol 1993;100(5):633–9.
30. Stavri GT, Hong Y, Zachary IC, et al. Hypoxia and platelet-derived growth factor-BB synergistically upregulate the expression of vascular endothelial growth factor in vascular smooth muscle cells. FEBS Lett 1995;358(3):311–5.
31. Lindahl P, Johansson BR, Leveen P, et al. Pericyte loss and microaneurysm formation in PDGF-B-deficient mice. Science 1997;277(5323):242–5.
32. Sundberg C, Branting M, Gerdin B, et al. Tumor cell and connective tissue cell interactions in human colorectal adenocarcinoma. Transfer of platelet-derived growth factor-AB/BB to stromal cells. Am J Pathol 1997;151(2):479–92.
33. Grotendorst GR, Martin GR, Pencev D, et al. Stimulation of granulation tissue formation by platelet-derived growth factor in normal and diabetic rats. J Clin Invest 1985;76(6):2323–9.

34. Pierce GF, Mustoe TA, Senior RM, et al. In vivo incisional wound healing augmented by platelet-derived growth factor and recombinant c-sis gene homodimeric proteins. J Exp Med 1988;167(3):974–87.

35. Pierce GF, Mustoe TA, Lingelbach J, et al. Platelet-derived growth factor and transforming growth factor-beta enhance tissue repair activities by unique mechanisms. J Cell Biol 1989;109(1):429–40.

36. Sprugel KH, McPherson JM, Clowes AW, et al. Effects of growth factors in vivo. I. Cell ingrowth into porous subcutaneous chambers. Am J Pathol 1987;129(3): 601–13.

37. Mustoe TA, Pierce GF, Morishima C, et al. Growth factor-induced acceleration of tissue repair through direct and inductive activities in a rabbit dermal ulcer model. J Clin Invest 1991;87(2):694–703.

38. Pierce GF, Veande Berg J, Rudolph R, et al. Platelet-derived growth factor-BB and transforming growth factor beta 1 selectively modulate glycosaminoglycans, collagen, and myofibroblasts in excisional wounds. Am J Pathol 1991; 138(3):629–46.

39. Robson MC, Phillips LG, Thomason A, et al. Platelet-derived growth factor BB for the treatment of chronic pressure ulcers. Lancet 1992;339(8784):23–5.

40. Lynch SE, Colvin RB, Antoniades HN. Growth factors in wound healing. Single and synergistic effects on partial thickness porcine skin wounds. J Clin Invest 1989;84(2):640–6.

41. Greenhalgh DG, Hummel RP, Albertson S, et al. Synergistic actions of platelet-derived growth factor and the insulin-like growth factors in vivo. Wound Repair Regen 1993;1(2):69–81.

42. Brown RL, Breeden MP, Greenhalgh DG. PDGF and TGF-alpha act synergistically to improve wound healing in the genetically diabetic mouse. J Surg Res 1994;56(6):562–70.

43. Mustoe TA, Purdy J, Gramates P, et al. Reversal of impaired wound healing in irradiated rats by platelet-derived growth factor-BB. Am J Surg 1989;158(4): 345–50.

44. Greenhalgh DG, Sprugel KH, Murray MJ, et al. PDGF and FGF stimulate wound healing in the genetically diabetic mouse. Am J Pathol 1990;136(6):1235–46.

45. Uhl E, Rosken F, Sirsjo A, et al. Influence of platelet-derived growth factor on microcirculation during normal and impaired wound healing. Wound Repair Regen 2003;11(5):361–7.

46. Lepisto J, Laato M, Miinikoski J, et al. Effects of homodimeric isoforms of platelet-derived growth factor (PDGF-AA and PDGF-BB) on wound healing in rat. J Surg Res 1992;53(6):596–601.

47. Deuel TF, Kawahara RS, Mustoe TA, et al. Growth factors and wound healing: platelet-derived growth factor as a model cytokine. Annu Rev Med 1991;42: 567–84.

48. Sprugel KH, Greenhalgh DG, Murray MJ, et al. Platelet-derived growth factor and impaired wound healing. Prog Clin Biol Res 1991;365:327–40.

49. Doxey DL, Ng MC, Dill RE, et al. Platelet derived growth factor levels in wounds in diabetic rates. Life Sci 1995;57(11):1111–23.

50. Embil JM, Papp K, Sibbald G, et al. Recombinant human platelet-derived growth factor-BB (becaplermin) for healing chronic lower extremity diabetic ulcers: an open-label clinical evaluation of efficacy. Wound Repair Regen 2000;8(3):162–8.

51. Smiell JM, Wieman TJ, Steed DL, et al. Efficacy and safety of becaplermin (recombinant human platelet-derived growth factor-BB) in patients with nonhealing,

lower extremity diabetic ulcers: a combined analysis of four randomized studies. Wound Repair Regen 1999;7(5):335–46.

52. Steed DL. Clinical evaluation of recombinant human platelet-derived growth factor for the treatment of lower extremity diabetic ulcers. Diabetic Ulcer Study Group. J Vasc Surg 1995;21(1):71–8.

53. Rees RS, Robson MC, Smiell JM, et al. Becaplermin gel in the treatment of pressure ulcers: a phase II randomized, double-blind, placebo-controlled study. Wound Repair Regen 1999;7(3):141–7.

54. Wieman TJ, Smiell JM, Su Y. Efficacy and safety of a topical gel formulation of recombinant human platelet-derived growth factor-BB (becaplermin) in patients with chronic neuropathic diabetic ulcers. A phase III randomized placebo-controlled double-blind study. Diabetes Care 1998;21(5):822–7.

55. Andrew JG, Hoyland JA, Freemont AJ, et al. Platelet-derived growth factor expression in normally healing human fractures. Bone 1995;16(4):455–60.

56. Nash TJ, Howlett CR, Martin C, et al. Effect of platelet-derived growth factor on tibial osteotomies in rabbits. Bone 1994;15(2):203–8.

57. Wahl SM, Hunt DA, Wakefield LM, et al. Transforming growth factor type beta induces monocyte chemotaxis and growth factor production. Proc Natl Acad Sci U S A 1987;84(16):5788–92.

58. Lawrence W, Diegelmann R. Growth factors in wound healing. Clin Dermatol 1994;12(1):157–69.

59. Sporn MB, Roberts AB, Wakefield LM, et al. Transforming growth factor-beta: biological function and chemical structure. Science 1986;233(4763):532–4.

60. Bassols A, Massague J. Transforming growth factor beta regulates the expression and structure of extracellular chondroitin/dermatan sulfate proteoglycans. J Biol Chem 1988;263(6):3039–45.

61. Fukamizu J, Grinnell F. Spatial organization of extracellular matrix and fibroblast activity: effects of serum, TGF-Beta and Fibronectin. Exp Cell Res 1990;190(2):276–82.

62. Goldberg MT, Han YP, Yan C, et al. TNF-alpha suppresses alpha-smooth muscle actin expression in human dermal fibroblasts: an implication for abnormal wound healing. J Invest Dermatol 2007;127(11):2645–55.

63. Greenwel P, Inagaki Y, Hu W, et al. Sp1 is required for the early response of alpha2(I) collagen to transforming growth factor-beta1. J Biol Chem 1997;272(32):19738–45.

64. Mauviel A, Chung KY, Agarwal A, et al. Cell-specific induction of distinct oncogenes of the Jun family is responsible for differential regulation of collagenase gene expression by transforming growth factor-beta in fibroblasts and keratinocytes. J Biol Chem 1996;271(18):10917–23.

65. Papakonstantinou E, Aletras AJ, Roth M, et al. Hypoxia modulates the effects of transforming growth factor-beta isoforms on matrix-formation by primary human lung fibroblasts. Cytokine 2003;24(1–2):25–35.

66. Riedel K, Riedel F, Goessler UR, et al. TGF-beta antisense therapy increases angiogenic potential in human keratinocytes in vitro. Arch Med Res 2007;38(1):45–51.

67. Ignotz R, Endo T, Massague J. Regulation of fibronectin and type I collagen mRNA levels by transforming growth factor-beta. J Biol Chem 1987;262(14):6443–6.

68. Meckmongkol TT, Harmon R, McKeown-Longo P, et al. The fibronectin synergy site modulates TGF-beta-dependent fibroblast contraction. Biochem Biophys Res Commun 2007;360(4):709–14.

69. Cordeiro MF, Reichel MB, Gay JA, et al. Transforming growth factor-beta1, -beta2, and -beta3 in vivo: effects on normal and mitomycin C-modulated conjunctival scarring. Invest Ophthalmol Vis Sci 1999;40(9):1975–82.
70. Roberts AB, Sporn MB, Assoian RK, et al. Transforming growth factor type beta: rapid induction of fibrosis and angiogenesis in vivo and stimulation of collagen formation in vitro. Proc Natl Acad Sci U S A 1986;83(12):4167–71.
71. Zeng G, McCue HM, Mastrangelo L, et al. Endogenous TGF-beta activity is modified during cellular aging: effects on metalloproteinase and TIMP-1 expression. Exp Cell Res 1996;228(2):271–6.
72. Robey PG, Young MF, Flanders KC, et al. Osteoblasts synthesize and respond to transforming growth factor-type beta (TGF-beta) in vitro. J Cell Biol 1987;105(1): 457–63.
73. Lieberman JR, Daluiski A, Einhorn TA. The role of growth factors in the repair of bone: biology and clinical applications. J Bone Joint Surg Am 2002;84-A(6): 1032–44.
74. Bolander ME. Regulation of fracture repair by growth factors. Proc Soc Exp Biol Med 1992;200(2):165–70.
75. Joyce ME, Jingushi S, Bolander ME. Transforming growth factor-beta in the regulation of fracture repair. Orthop Clin North Am 1990;21(1):199–209.
76. Bourque WT, Gross MT, Hall BK. Expression of four growth factors during fracture repair. Int J Dev Biol 1993;37(4):573–9.
77. Grageda E. Platelet-rich plasma and bone graft materials: a review and a standardized research protocol. Implant Dent 2004;13(4):301–9.
78. Lind M, Schumacker B, Søballe K, et al. Transforming growth factor-beta enhances fracture healing in rabbit tibiae. Acta Orthop Scand 1993;64(5):553–6.
79. Nielsen HM, Andreassen TT, Ledet T, et al. Local injection of TGF-beta increases the strength of tibial fractures in the rat. Acta Orthop Scand 1994;65(1):37–41.
80. Critchlow MA, Bland YS, Ashhurst DE. The effect of exogenous transforming growth factor-beta 2 on healing fractures in the rabbit. Bone 1995;16(5):521–7.
81. Beck LS, Amento EP, Xu Y, et al. TGF-beta 1 induces bone closure of skull defects: temporal dynamics of bone formation in defects exposed to rhTGF-beta 1. J Bone Miner Res 1993;8(6):753–61.
82. Beck LS, Deguzman L, Lee WP, et al. Rapid publication. TGF-beta 1 induces bone closure of skull defects. J Bone Miner Res 1991;6(11):1257–65.
83. Nanney LB, Magid M, Stoscheck CM, et al. Comparison of epidermal growth factor binding and receptor distribution in normal human epidermis and epidermal appendages. J Invest Dermatol 1984;83(5):385–93.
84. Nanney LB, McKanna JA, Stoscheck CM, et al. Visualization of epidermal growth factor receptors in human epidermis. J Invest Dermatol 1984;82(2): 165–9.
85. Grotendorst G, Soma Y, Takehara K, et al. EGF and TGF-alpha are potent chemoattractants for endothelial cells and EGF-like peptides are present at sites of tissue regeneration. J Clin Invest 1989;139(3):617–23.
86. Tokumaru S, Higashiyama S, Endo T, et al. Ectodomain shedding of epidermal growth factor receptor ligands is required for keratinocyte migration in cutaneous wound healing. J Cell Biol 2000;151(2):209–20.
87. Nanney LB. Epidermal and dermal effects of epidermal growth factor during wound repair. J Invest Dermatol 1990;94(5):624–9.
88. Reiss M, Sartorelli AC. Regulation of growth and differentiation of human keratinocytes by type beta transforming growth factor and epidermal growth factor. Cancer Res 1987;47(24 Pt 1):6705–9.

89. Brown GL, Nanney LB, Griffen J, et al. Enhancement of wound healing by topical treatment with epidermal growth factor. N Engl J Med 1989;321(2):76–9.

90. Falanga V, Eaglstein WH, Bucalo B, et al. Topical use of human recombinant epidermal growth factor (h-EGF) in venous ulcers. J Dermatol Surg Oncol 1992;18(7):604–6.

91. Viswanathan V, Pendsey S, Sekar N, et al. A Phase III Study to Evaluate the Safety and Efficacy of Recombinant Human Epidermal Growth Factor (REGEN-D™ 150) in Healing Diabetic foot ulcers. Wounds 2006;18(7):186–96.

92. Grant M, Jerdan J, Merimee T. Insulin-like growth factor-I modulates endothelial cell chemotaxis. J Clin Endocrinol Metab 1987;65(2):370–1.

93. Clemmons DR, Maile LA, Ling Y, et al. Role of the integrin alphaVbeta3 in mediating increased smooth muscle cell responsiveness to IGF-I in response to hyperglycemic stress. Growth Horm IGF Res 2007;17(4):265–70.

94. Panagakos FS. Insulin-like growth factors-I and -II stimulate chemotaxis of osteoblasts isolated from fetal rat calvaria. Biochimie 1993;75(11):991–4.

95. Lynch SE, Nixon JC, Colvin RB, et al. Role of platelet derived growth factors in wound healing: synergistic effects with other growth factors. Proc Natl Acad Sci U S A 1987;84(21):7696–700.

96. Guvakova MA. Insulin-like growth factors control cell migration in health and disease. Int J Biochem Cell Biol 2007;39(5):890–909.

97. Clemens TL, Chernausek SD. Genetic strategies for elucidating insulin-like growth factor action in bone. Growth Horm IGF Res 2004;14(3):195–9.

98. Niu T, Rosen CJ. The insulin-like growth factor-I gene and osteoporosis: a critical appraisal. Gene 2005;361:38–56.

99. Canalis E, Rydziel S, Delany AM, et al. Insulin-like growth factors inhibit interstitial collagenase synthesis in bone cell cultures. Endocrinology 1995;136(4):1348–54.

100. Jonsson KB, Ljunghall S, Karlström O, et al. Insulin-like growth factor 1 enhances the formation of type 1 collagen in hydrocortisone-treated human osteoblasts. Biosci Rep 1993;13(5):297–302.

101. Mohan S, Baylink DJ. Insulin-like growth factor system components and the coupling of bone formation to resorption. Horm Res 1996;45(Suppl 1):59–62.

102. Rosen CJ, Hunter LR, Donahue SJ. Insulin-like growth factors and bone: the osteoporosis connection revisited. Proc Soc Exp Biol Med 1994;206(2):83–102.

103. Eingartner C, Coerper s, Fritz J, et al. Growth factors in distraction osteogenesis. Immuno-histological pattern of TGF-beta1 and IGF-I in human callus induced by distraction osteogenesis. Int Orthop 1999;23(5):253–9.

104. Okazaki K, Jingushi S, Ikenoue T, et al. Expression of parathyroid hormone-related peptide and insulin-like growth factor I during rat fracture healing. J Orthop Res 2003;21(3):511–20.

105. Bak B, Jorgensen PH, Andreassen TT. Dose response of growth hormone on fracture healing in the rat. Acta Orthop Scand 1990;61(1):54–7.

106. Andrew JG, Hoyland J, Freemont AJ, et al. Insulinlike growth factor gene expression in human fracture callus. Calcif Tissue Int 1993;53(2):97–102.

107. Schmidmaier G, Wildemann B, Bail H, et al. Local application of growth factors (insulin-like growth factor-1 and transforming growth factor-beta1) from a biodegradable poly(D, L-lactide) coating of osteosynthetic implants accelerates fracture healing in rats. Bone 2001;28(4):341–50.

108. Thaller SR, Dart A, Tesluk H. The effects of insulin-like growth factor-1 on critical-size calvarial defects in Sprague-Dawley rats. Ann Plast Surg 1993;31(5):429–33.

109. Raschke M, Wildemann B, Inden P, et al. Insulinlike growth factor-1 and transforming growth factor-beta1 accelerates osteotomy healing using polylactide-coated implants as a delivery system: a biomechanical and histological study in minipigs. Bone 2002;30(1):144–51.

110. Fowlkes JL, Thrailkill KM, Liu L, et al. Effects of systemic and local administration of recombinant human IGF-I (rhIGF-I) on de novo bone formation in an aged mouse model. J Bone Miner Res 2006;21(9):1359–66.

111. Zhou H, Dong Q, Zhou X, et al. Calvarial defects repair in nude mice by human bone marrow mesenchymal stem cells transfected with insulin like growth factor-1. Bone 2008;43:S60.

112. Banks RE, Forbes MA, Kinsey SE, et al. Release of angiogenic cytokine vascular endothelial growth factor (VEGF) from platelets: significance for VEGF in cancer biology. Br J Cancer 1998;77(6):956–64.

113. Thomas KA. Vascular endothelial growth factor, a potent and selective angiogenic agent. J Biol Chem 1996;271(2):603–6.

114. Breier G, Damert A, Plate KH, et al. Angiogenesis in embryos and ischemic diseases. Thromb Haemost 1997;78(1):678–83.

115. Olander JV, Connolly DT, DeLarco JE. Specific binding of vascular permeability factor to endothelial cells. Biochem Biophys Res Commun 1991; 175(1):68–76.

116. Peters KG, De Vries C, Williams LT. Vascular endothelial growth factor receptor expression during embryogenesis and tissue repair suggests a role in endothelial differentiation and blood vessel growth. Proc Natl Acad Sci U S A 1993; 90(19):8915–9.

117. Yebra M, Parry GC, Strömblad S, et al. Requirement of receptor-bound urokinase-type plasminogen activator for integrin alphavbeta5-directed cell migration. J Biol Chem 1996;271(46):29393–9.

118. Suzuma K, Takagi H, Otani A, et al. Hypoxia and vascular endothelial growth factor stimulate angiogenic integrin expression in bovine retinal microvascular endothelial cells. Invest Opthalmol Vis Sci 1998;39(6):1028–35.

119. Senger DR, Ledbetter SR, Claffey KP, et al. Stimulation of endothelial cell migration by vascular permeability factor/vascular endothelial growth factor through cooperative mechanisms involving the alphavbeta3 integrin, osteopontin, and thrombin. Am J Pathol 1996;149(1):293–305.

120. Pepper MS, Ferrara N, Orci L, et al. Potent synergism between vascular endothelial growth factor and basic fibroblast growth factor in the induction of angiogenesis in vitro. Biochem Biophys Res Commun 1992;189(2): 824–31.

121. Watanabe Y, Lee SW, Detmar M, et al. Vascular permeability factor/vascular endothelial growth factor (VPF/VEGF) delays and induces escape from senescence in human dermal microvascular endothelial cells. Oncogene 1997; 14(17):2025–32.

122. Hong YK, Lange-Asschenfeldt B, Velasco P, et al. VEGF-A promotes tissue repair-associated lymphatic vessel formation via VEGFR-2 and the alpha1beta1 and alpha2- beta1 integrins. FASEB J 2004;18(10):1111–3.

123. Walder CE, Errett CJ, Bunting S, et al. Vascular endothelial growth factor augments muscle blood flow and function in a rabbit model of chronic hindlimb ischemia. J Cardiovasc Pharmacol 1996;27(1):91–8.

124. Bauters C, Asahara T, Zheng LP, et al. Site-specific therapeutic angiogenesis after systemic administration of vascular endothelial growth factor. J Vasc Surg 1995;21(2):314–24.

125. Bauters C, Asahara T, Zheng LP, et al. Physiological assessment of augmented vascularity induced by VEGF in ischemic rabbit hindlimb. Am J Phys 1994;267 (4 Pt 2):H1263–71.

126. Takeshita S, Pu LQ, Stein LA, et al. Intramuscular administration of vascular endothelial growth factor induces dose-dependent collateral artery augmentation in a rabbit model of chronic limb ischemia. Circulation 1994;90(5 Pt 2):II228–34.

127. Takeshita S, Zheng LP, Brogi E, et al. Therapeutic angiogenesis. A single intra-arterial bolus of vascular endothelial growth factor augments revascularization in a rabbit ischemic hind limb model. J Clin Invest 1994;93(2):662–70.

128. Galiano RD, Tepper OM, Pelo CR, et al. Topical vascular endothelial growth factor accelerates diabetic wound healing through increased angiogenesis and by mobilizing and recruiting bone marrow-derived cells. Am J Pathol 2004;164(6):1935–47.

129. Baumgartner I, Pieczek A, Manor O, et al. Constitutive expression of phVEGF165 after intramuscular gene transfer promotes collateral vessel development in patients with critical limb ischemia. Circulation 1998;97(12):1114–23.

130. Nagy JA, Vasile E, Feng D, et al. Vascular permeability factor/vascular endothelial growth factor induces lymphangiogenesis as well as angiogenesis. J Exp Med 2002;196(11):1497–506.

131. Carmeliet P VEGF. gene therapy: stimulating angiogenesis or angioma-genesis? Nat Med 2000;6(10):1102–3.

132. Maes C, Carmeliet P, Moermans K, et al. Impaired angiogenesis and endochondral bone formation in mice lacking the vascular endothelial growth factor isoforms VEGF164 and VEGF188. Mech Dev 2002;111(1–2):61–73.

133. Slater M, Patava J, Kingham K, et al. Involvement of platelets in stimulating osteogenic activity. J Orthop Res 1995;13(5):655–63.

134. Lowery GL, Kulkarni S, Pennisi AE. Use of autologous growth factors in lumbar spinal fusion. Bone 1999;25(2 Suppl):47S–50S.

135. Whitman DH, Berry RL, Green DM. Platelet gel: an autologous alternative to fibrin glue with applications in oral and maxillofacial surgery. J Oral Maxillofac Surg 1997;55(11):1294–9.

136. Marx RE, Carlson ER, Eichstaedt RM, et al. Platelet-rich plasma: growth factor enhancement for bone grafts. Oral Surg Oral Med Oral Pathol Oral Radiol Endod 1998;85(6):638–46.

137. Kevy SV, Jacobson MS. Comparison of methods for point of care preparation of autologous platelet gel. J Extra Corpor Technol 2004;36(1):28–35.

138. Margolis DJ, Kantor J, Santanna J, et al. Effectiveness of platelet releasate for the treatment of diabetic neuropathic foot ulcers. Diabetes Care 2001;24(3): 483–8.

139. Crovetti G, Martinelli G, Issi M, et al. Platelet gel for healing cutaneous chronic wounds. Transfus Apheresis Sci 2004;30(2):145–51.

140. Eppley BL. Platelet rich plasma: a review of biology and applications in plastic surgery. Plast Reconstr Surg 2006;118(6):147e–59e.

141. Gonshor A. Technique for producing platelet rich plasma and platelet concentrate: background and process. Int J Periodontics Restorative Dent 2002; 22(6):547–57.

142. Gandhi A, Doumas C, O'Connor JP, et al. The effects of local platelet rich plasma delivery on diabetic fracture healing. Bone 2006;38(4):540–6.

143. Man D, Plosker H, Winland-Brown JE. The use of autologous platelet-rich plasma (platelet gel) and autologous platelet-poor plasma (fibrin glue) in cosmetic surgery. Plast Reconstr Surg 2001;107(1):229–37.

144. Petrungaro PS. Using platelet-rich plasma to accelerate soft tissue maturation in esthetic periodontal surgery. Compend Contin Educ Dent 2001;22(9):729–32.
145. Siebrecht MAN, De Rooij PP, Arm DM, et al. Platelet concentrate increases bone ingrowth into porous hydroxyapatite. Orthopedics 2002;25:169–72.
146. Marlovits S, Mousavi M, Gäbler C, et al. A new simplified technique for producing platelet-rich plasma: A short technical note. Eur Spine J 2004; 13(Suppl 1):S102–6.
147. Lozada JL, Caplanis N, Proussaefs P, et al. Platelet-rich plasma application in sinus graft surgery: Part I. Background and processing techniques. J Oral Implantol 2001;27(1):38–42.
148. Gandhi A, Bibbo C, Pinzur M, et al. The role of platelet-rich plasma in foot and ankle surgery. Foot Ankle Clin 2005;10(4):621–37.
149. Landesberg R, Roy M, Glickman RS. Quantification of growth factor levels using a simplified method of platelet-rich plasma gel preparation. J Oral Maxillofac Surg 2000;58(3):297–300.
150. Efeoglu C, Akçay YD, Ertürk S. A modified method of preparing platelet-rich plasma: an experimental study. J Oral Maxillofac Surg 2004;62(11):1403–7.
151. Roukis TS, Zgonis T, Tiernan B. Autologous platelet-rich plasma for wound and osseous healing: a review of the literature and commercially available products. Adv Ther 2006;23(2):218–37.
152. Weibrich G, Kleis WK, Hitzler WE, et al. Comparison of the platelet concentrate collection system with the plasma-rich-in-growth-factors kit to produce platelet-rich plasma: a technical report. Int J Oral Maxillofac Implants 2005;20(1):118–23.
153. Weibrich G, Hansen T, Kleis W, et al. Effect of platelet concentration in platelet-rich plasma on peri-implant bone regeneration. Bone 2004;34(4):665–71.
154. Zimmermann R, Arnold D, Strasser E, et al. Sample preparation technique and white cell content influence the detectable levels of growth factors in platelet concentrates. Vox Sang 2003;85(4):283–9.
155. Anderson NA, Pamphilon DH, Tandy NJ, et al. Comparison of platelet-rich plasma collection using the Haemonetics PCS and Baxter Autopheresis C. Vox Sang 1991;60(3):155–8.
156. Christie RJ, Carrington L, Alving B. Postoperative bleeding induced by topical bovine thrombin: report of two cases. Surgery 1997;121(6):708–10.
157. Rapaport SI, Zivelin A, Minow RA, et al. Clinical significance of antibodies to bovine and human thrombin and factor V after surgical use of bovine thrombin. Am J Pathol 1992;97(1):84–91.
158. Zehnder JL, Leung LL. Development of antibodies to thrombin and factor V with recurrent bleeding in a patient exposed to topical bovine thrombin. Blood 1990; 76(10):2011–6.
159. Fennis JP, Stoelinga PJ, Jansen JA. Mandibular reconstruction: a clinical and radiographic animal study on the use of autogenous scaffolds and platelet-rich plasma. Int J Oral Maxillofac Surg 2002;31(3):281–6.
160. Arpornmaeklong P, Kochel M, Depprich R, et al. Influence of platelet-rich plasma (PRP) on osteogenic differentiation of rat bone marrow stromal cells. An in vitro study. Int J Oral Maxillofac Implants 2004;33(1):60–70.
161. Slapnicka J, Fassmann A, Strasak L, et al. Effects of activated and nonactivated platelet-rich plasma on proliferation of human osteoblasts in vitro. J Oral Maxillofac Surg 2008;66(2):297–301.
162. Lucarelli E, Beccheroni A, Donati D, et al. Platelet-derived growth factors enhance proliferation of human stromal stem cells. Biomaterials 2003;24(18): 3095–100.

163. Kanno T, Takahashi T, Tsujisawa T, et al. Platelet-rich plasma enhances human osteoblast-like cell proliferation and differentiation. J Oral Maxillofac Surg 2005;63(3):362–9.

164. Tomoyasu A, Higashio K, Kanomata K, et al. Platelet-rich plasma stimulates osteoblastic differentiation in the presence of BMPs. Biochem Biophys Res Commun 2007;361(1):62–7.

165. Ranly DM, Lohmann CH, Andreacchio D, et al. Platelet-rich plasma inhibits demineralized bone matrix-induced bone formation in nude mice. J Bone Joint Surg 2007;89-A(1):139–47.

166. Ranly DM, McMillan J, Keller T, et al. Platelet-derived growth factor inhibits demineralized bone matrix-induced intramuscular cartilage and bone formation. A study of immunocompromised mice. J Bone Joint Surg Am 2005;87-A(9): 2052–64.

167. Butterfield KJ, Bennett J, Gronowicz G, et al. Effect of platelet-rich plasma with autogenous bone graft for maxillary sinus augmentation in a rabbit model. J Oral Maxillofac Surg 2005;63(3):370–6.

168. Kim ES, Park EJ, Choung PH. Platelet concentration and its effect on bone formation in calvarial defects: an experimental study in rabbits. J Prosthet Dent 2001;86(4):428–33.

169. Kasten P, Vogel J, Geiger F, et al. The effect of platelet-rich plasma on healing in critical-size long-bone defects. Biomaterials 2008;29(29):3983–92.

170. Kroese-Deutman HC, Vehof JW, Spauwen PH, et al. Orthotopic bone formation in titanium fiber mesh loaded with platelet-rich plasma and placed in segmental defects. Int J Oral Maxillofac Implants 2008;37(6):542–9.

171. Aghaloo TL, Moy PK, Freymiller EG. Evaluation of platelet-rich plasma in combination with freeze-dried bone in the rabbit cranium. A pilot study. Clin Oral Implants Res 2005;16(2):250–7.

172. Aghaloo TL, Moy PK, Freymiller EG. Evaluation of platelet-rich plasma in combination with anorganic bovine bone in the rabbit cranium: a pilot study. Int J Oral Maxillofac Implants 2004;19(1):59–65.

173. Aghaloo TL, Moy PK, Freymiller EG. Investigation of platelet-rich plasma in rabbit cranial defects: A pilot study. J Oral Maxillofac Surg 2002;60(10): 1176–81.

174. Thorwarth M, Rupprecht S, Falk S, et al. Expression of bone matrix proteins during de novo bone formation using a bovine collagen and platelet-rich plasma (PRP)–an immunohistochemical analysis. Biomaterials 2005;26(15):2575–84.

175. Wiltfang J, Kloss FR, Kessler P, et al. Effects of platelet-rich plasma on bone healing in combination with autogenous bone and bone substitutes in critical-size defects. An animal experiment. Clin Oral Implants Res 2004;15(2): 187–93.

176. Schlegel KA, Donath K, Rupprecht S, et al. De novo bone formation using bovine collagen and platelet-rich plasma. Biomaterials 2004;25(23):5387–93.

177. Klongnoi B, Rupprecht S, Kessler P, et al. Lack of beneficial effects of platelet-rich plasma on sinus augmentation using a fluorhydroxyapatite or autogenous bone: an explorative study. J Clin Periodontol 2006;33(7):500–9.

178. Roldán JC, Knueppel H, Schmidt C, et al. Single-stage sinus augmentation with cancellous iliac bone and anorganic bovine bone in the presence of platelet-rich plasma in the miniature pig. Clin Oral Implants Res 2008;19(4):373–8.

179. Mooren RE, Merkx MA, Bronkhorst EM, et al. The effect of platelet-rich plasma on early and late bone healing: an experimental study in goats. Int J Oral Maxillofac Surg 2007;36(7):626–31.

180. Jensen TB, Rahbek O, Overgaard S, et al. Platelet rich plasma and fresh frozen bone allograft as enhancement of implant fixation. An experimental study in dogs. J Orthop Res 2004;22(3):653–8.
181. Jensen TB, Rahbek O, Overgaard S, et al. No effect of platelet-rich plasma with frozen or processed bone allograft around noncemented implants. Int Orthop 2005;29(2):67–72.
182. Choi BH, Im CJ, Huh JY, et al. Effect of platelet-rich plasma on bone regeneration in autogenous bone graft. Int J Oral Maxillofac Implants 2004;33(1):56–9.
183. Sarkar MR, Augat P, Shefelbine SJ, et al. Bone formation in a long bone defect model using a platelet-rich plasma-loaded collagen scaffold. Biomaterials 2006; 27(9):1817–23.
184. Robiony M, Polini F, Costa F, et al. Osteogenesis distraction and platelet-rich plasma for bone restoration of the severely atrophic mandible: preliminary results. J Oral Maxillofac Surg 2002;60(6):630–5.
185. Kassolis JD, Reynolds MA. Evaluation of the adjunctive benefits of platelet-rich plasma in subantral sinus augmentation. J Craniofac Surg 2005;16(2):280–7.
186. Kassolis JD, Rosen PS, Reynolds MA. Alveolar ridge and sinus augmentation utilizing platelet-rich plasma in combination with freeze-dried bone allograft: case series. J Periodontol 2000;71(10):1654–61.
187. Maiorana C, Sommariva L, Brivio P, et al. Maxillary sinus augmentation with anorganic bovine bone (Bio-Oss) and autologous platelet-rich plasma: preliminary clinical and histologic evaluations. Int J Periodontics Restorative Dent 2003; 23(3):227–35.
188. Rodriguez A, Anastassov GE, Lee H, et al. Maxillary sinus augmentation with deproteinated bovine bone and platelet rich plasma with simultaneous insertion of endosseous implants. J Oral Maxillofac Surg 2003;61(2):157–63.
189. Consolo U, Zaffe D, Bertoldi C, et al. Platelet-rich plasma activity on maxillary sinus floor augmentation by autologous bone. Clin Oral Implants Res 2007; 18(2):252–62.
190. Thor A, Franke-Stenport V, Johansson CB, et al. Early bone formation in human bone grafts treated with platelet-rich plasma: preliminary histomorphometric results. Int J Oral Maxillofac Surg 2007;36(12):1164–71.
191. Dawson J, Thorogood M, Marks SA, et al. The prevalence of foot problems in older women: a cause for concern. J Public Health Med 2002;24(2):77–84.
192. Schaaf H, Streckbein P, Lendeckel S, et al. Topical use of platelet-rich plasma to influence bone volume in maxillary augmentation: a prospective randomized trial. Vox Sang 2008;94(1):64–9.
193. Schaaf H, Streckbein P, Lendeckel S, et al. Sinus lift augmentation using autogenous bone grafts and platelet-rich plasma: radiographic results. Oral Surg Oral Med Oral Pathol Oral Radiol Endod 2008;106(5):673–8.
194. Kitoh H, Kitakoji T, Tsuchiya H, et al. Distraction osteogenesis of the lower extremity in patients with achondroplasia/hypochondroplasia treated with transplantation of culture-expanded bone marrow cells and platelet-rich plasma. J Pediatr Orthop 2007;27(6):629–34.
195. Kitoh H, Kitakoji T, Tsuchiya H, et al. Transplantation of culture expanded bone marrow cells and platelet rich plasma in distraction osteogenesis of the long bones. Bone 2007;40(2):522–8.
196. Kitoh H, Kitakoji T, Tsuchiya H, et al. Transplantation of marrow-derived mesenchymal stem cells and platelet-rich plasma during distraction osteogenesis—a preliminary result of three cases. Bone 2004;35(4):892–8.

197. Castro FPJ. Role of activated growth factors in lumbar spinal fusions. J Spinal Disord Tech 2004;17(5):380–4.
198. Carreon LY, Glassman SD, Anekstein Y, et al. Platelet gel (AGF) fails to increase fusion rates in instrumented posterolateral fusions. Spine 2005;30(9):E243–6.
199. Jenis LG, Banco RJ, Kwon B. A prospective study of autologous growth factors (AGF) in lumbar interbody. Spine J 2006;6(1):14–20.
200. Weiner BK, Walker M. Efficacy of autologous growth factors in lumbar intertransverse fusions. Spine 2003;28(17):1968–70.
201. Mariconda M, Cozzolino F, Cozzolino A, et al. Platelet gel supplementation in long bone nonunions treated by external fixation. J Orthop Trauma 2008; 22(5):342–5.
202. Coetzee JC, Pomeroy GC, Watts JD, et al. The use of autologous concentrated growth factors to promote syndesmosis fusion in the agility total ankle replacement. A preliminary study. Foot Ankle Int 2005;26(10):840–6.
203. Barrow CR, Pomeroy GC. Enhancement of syndesmotic fusion rates in total ankle arthroplasty with the use of autologous platelet concentrate. Foot Ankle Int 2005;26(6):458–61.
204. Bibbo C, Bono CM, Lin SS. Union rates using autologous platelet concentrate alone and with bone graft in high-risk foot and ankle surgery patients. J Surg Orthop Adv 2005;14(1):17–22.
205. Grant WP, Jerlin EA, Pietrzak WS, et al. The utilization of autologous growth factors for the facilitation of fusion in complex neuropathic fractures in the diabetic population. Clin Podiatr Med Surg 2005;22(4):561–84.
206. Boc SF, D'Angelantonio A, Grant S. The triplane Austin bunionectomy: A review and retrospective analysis. J Foot Ankle Surg 1991;30(4):375–82.
207. Kakudo N, Minakata T, Mitsui T, et al. Proliferation-promoting effect of platelet-rich plasma on human adipose-derived stem cells and human dermal fibroblasts. Plast Reconstr Surg 2008;122(5):1352–60.
208. Graziani F, Ivanovski S, Cei S, et al. The in vitro effect of different PRP concentrations on osteoblasts and fibroblasts. Clin Oral Implants Res 2006;17(2): 212–9.
209. Lundquist R, Dziegiel MH, Agren MS. Bioactivity and stability of endogenous fibrogenic factors in platelet-rich fibrin. Wound Repair Regen 2008;16(3):356–63.
210. Phillips GD, Stone AM, Whitehead RA, et al. Platelet derived wound healing factors (PDWHF) accelerate and augment wound healing angiogenesis in the rat. Vivo 1994;8(2):167–71.
211. Tanaka R, Ichioka S, Sekiya N, et al. Elastic plasma protein film blended with platelet releasate accelerates healing of diabetic mouse skin wounds. Vox Sang 2007;93(1):49–56.
212. Ito H, Shimizu A, Miyamoto T, et al. Clinical significance of increased mobility in the sagittal plane in patients with hallux valgus. Foot Ankle Int 1999;20(1): 29–32.
213. Moulin V, Lawny F, Barritault D, et al. Platelet releasate treatment improves skin healing in diabetic rats through endogenous growth factor secretion. Cell Mol Biol 1998;44(6):961–71.
214. Vermeulen P, Dickens S, Vranckx JJ. Platelet-rich plasma and keratinocytes enhance healing and deposition of fibronectin in a porcine full thickness wound model. J Plast Reconstr Aesthet Surg 2006;60(4):S14 (O43).
215. Carter CA, Jolly DG, Worden CES, et al. Platelet-rich plasma gel promotes differentiation and regeneration during equine wound healing. Exp Mol Pathol 2003; 74(3):244–55.

216. Chandra RK, Handorf C, West M, et al. Histologic effects of autologous platelet gel in skin flap healing. Arch Facial Plast Surg 2007;9(4):260–3.
217. Powell DM, Chang E, Farrior EH. Recovery from deep-plane rhytidectomy following unilateral wound treatment with autologous platelet gel. Arch Facial Plast Surg 2001;3(4):245–50.
218. Danielsen P, Jørgensen B, Karlsmark T, et al. Effect of topical autologous platelet-rich fibrin versus no intervention on epithelialization of donor sites and meshed split-thickness skin autografts: a randomized clinical trial. Plast Reconstr Surg 2008;122(5):1431–40.
219. Hom DB, Linzie BM, Huang TC. The healing effects of autologous platelet gel on acute human skin wounds. Arch Facial Plast Surg 2007;9(3):174–83.
220. Kazakos K, Lyras DN, Verettas D, et al. The use of autologous PRP gel as an aid in the management of acute trauma wounds. Injury 2009;40(8):801–5.
221. Doucette MM, Fylling C, Knighton DR. Amputation prevention in a high-risk population through comprehensive wound-healing protocol. Arch Phys Med Rehabil 1989;70(10):780–5.
222. Knighton DR, Fylling CP, Fiegel VD, et al. Amputation prevention in an independently reviewed at-risk diabetic population using a comprehensive wound care protocol. Am J Surg 1990;160(5):466–71.
223. Glover JL, Weingarten MS, Buchbinder DS, et al. A 4-year outcome-based retrospective study of wound healing and limb salvage in patients with chronic wounds. Adv Wound Care 1997;10(1):33–8.
224. Ganio C, Tenewitz FE, Wilson RC, et al. The treatment of chronic nonhealing wounds using autologous platelet-derived growth factors. J Foot Ankle Surg 1993;32(3):263–8.
225. Knighton DR, Ciresi KF, Fiegel VD, et al. Classification and treatment of chronic nonhealing wounds. Successful treatment with autologous platelet-derived wound healing factors (PDWHF). Ann Surg 1986;204(3):322–30.
226. Knighton DR, Ciresi K, Fiegel VD, et al. Stimulation of repair in chronic, nonhealing, cutaneous ulcers using platelet-derived wound healing formula. Surg Gynecol Obstet 1990;170(1):56–60.
227. Atri SC, Misra J, Bisht D, et al. Use of homologous platelet factors in achieving total healing of recalcitrant skin ulcers. Surgery 1990;108(3):508–12.
228. Steed DL, Goslen JB, Holloway GA, et al. Randomized prospective double-blind trial in healing chronic diabetic foot ulcers. CT-102 activated platelet supernatant, topical versus placebo. Diabetes Care 1992;15(11):1598–604.
229. Driver VR, Hanft J, Fylling CP, et al. A prospective, randomized, controlled trial of autologous platelet-rich plasma gel for the treatment of diabetic foot ulcers. Ostomy Wound Manage 2006;52(6):68–70, 72, 74.
230. Holloway GA, Steed DL, DeMarco JM, et al. A randomized controlled dose response trial of activated platelet supernatant, topical CT-102 in chronic, non-healing, diabetic wounds. WOUNDS 1993;5:160–8.
231. Krupski WC, Reilly LM, Perez S, et al. A prospective randomized trial of autologous platelet-derived wound healing factors for treatment of chronic nonhealing wounds: a preliminary report. J Vasc Surg 1991;14(4):526–32.
232. Akeda K, An HS, Okuma M, et al. Platelet-rich plasma stimulates porcine articular chondrocyte proliferation and matrix biosynthesis. Osteoarthr Cartil 2006; 14(12):1272–80.
233. Choi YC, Morris GM, Sokoloff L. Effect of platelet lysate on growth and sulfated glycosaminoglycan synthesis in articular chondrocyte cultures. Arthritis Rheum 1980;23(2):220–4.

234. Kaps C, Loch A, Haisch A, et al. Human platelet supernatant promotes proliferation but not differentiation of articular chondrocytes. Med Biol Eng Comput 2002;40(4):485–90.

235. Gaissmaier C, Fritz J, Krackhardt T, et al. Effect of human platelet supernatant on proliferation and matrix synthesis of human articular chondrocytes in monolayer and three-dimensional alginate cultures. Biomaterials 2005;26(14): 1953–60.

236. Saito M, Takahashi KA, Arai Y, et al. The preventative effect of platelet-rich plasma and biodegradable gelatin hydrogel microspheres on experimental osteoarthritis in the rabbit knee. Osteoarthr Cartil 2007;15(Suppl 3):C232.

237. Nakagawa K, Sasho T, Arai M, et al. Effects of autologous platelet-rich plasma on the metabolism of human articular chondrocytes. Osteoarthr Cartil 2007; 15(Suppl 2):B134.

238. de Mos M, van der Windt AE, Jahr H, et al. Can platelet-rich plasma enhance tendon repair? A cell culture study. Am J Sports Med 2008;36(6):1171–8.

239. Anitua E, Andía I, Sanchez M, et al. Autologous preparations rich in growth factors promote proliferation and induce VEGF and HGF production by human tendon cells in culture. J Orthop Res 2005;23(2):281–6.

240. Aspenberg P, Virchenko O. Platelet concentrate injection improves Achilles tendon repair in rats. Acta Orthop Scand 2004;75(1):93–9.

241. Virchenko O, Aspenberg P. How can one platelet injection after tendon injury lead to a stronger tendon after 4 weeks? Interplay between early regeneration and mechanical stimulation. Acta Orthop 2006;77(5):806–12.

242. Virchenko O, Grenegård M, Aspenberg P. Independent and additive stimulation of tendon repair by thrombin and platelets. Acta Orthop 2006;77(6):960–6.

243. Mishra A, Pavelko T. Treatment of chronic elbow tendinosis with buffered platelet-rich plasma. Am J Sports Med 2006;34(11):1774–8.

Bone Graft Substitutes and Allografts for Reconstruction of the Foot and Ankle

Emily A. Cook, DPM, MPH*, Jeremy J. Cook, DPM, MPH

KEYWORDS

- Bone graft substitute • Allograft • Xenograft
- Reconstruction • Foot • Ankle

It is estimated that more than 1,300,000 musculoskeletal bone grafts were distributed in the United States in 2005.[1] This is a clear indication that use of alternative bone grafting is often necessary, especially for reconstructive foot and ankle surgery. It is imperative that the foot and ankle surgeon acquire and maintain a fundamental understanding of alternative bone graft options. The surgeon should consider the purpose of the graft (eg, structural, filling in voids), the location of the graft, the local perfusion, the cost, and the potential graft advantages and limitations for each case. Patient factors, including comorbidities, body mass index (BMI), age, activity level, expectations, social determinants, and risk factors such as tobacco use, can also influence the graft choice.

BONE GRAFT CLASSIFICATION

The various types of bone grafts may be classified based on their primary material composition. Although many bone grafts consist of a composite of substances, they will usually contain 1 primary material. Therefore, it is easiest to remember each bone graft's basic properties so that it can be placed into 1 of these 6 basic categories (**Table 1**).

Regardless of the bone graft base material, it may be available in many shapes, sizes, and forms. In special circumstances, some grafts may be mixed with other substances, such as antibiotics. A graft may be structural, indicating that it is a solid piece of cortical, cancellous, or corticocancellous bone. The structural graft may or may not be machined and can be supplied as bulk graft. There are many forms of graft used for filling a void. They include

---

Department of Surgery, Division of Podiatric Surgery, Harvard Medical School, Beth Israel Deaconess Medical Center, One Deaconess Road, Boston, MA 02215, USA
* Corresponding author.
E-mail address: ecook@bidmc.harvard.edu (E. A. Cook).

Clin Podiatr Med Surg 26 (2009) 589–605
doi:10.1016/j.cpm.2009.07.003
podiatric.theclinics.com
0891-8422/09/$ – see front matter © 2009 Elsevier Inc. All rights reserved.

Table 1
Bone graft classification

Classification	Definition	Types
Autogenous bone grafts	Bone is transferred within the same person; considered gold-standard	Iliac crest, fibular, tibia, calcaneus
Allografts	Bone is transferred from one person to another (usually cadaveric)	Fresh, frozen and fresh-frozen, freeze-dried (lyophilized), demineralized
Xenografts	Bone is transferred between species	Bovine, equine
Synthetic bone grafts	Product is manufactured from synthetic materials	Calcium (calcium sulfate, calcium phosphate)
Factor-based bone grafts	Growth factors that are added to various carriers	Bone morphogenic protein, platelet-derived growth factor
Cell-based bone grafts	Live cells are added to various carriers	Mesenchymal stem cells

- Chips
- Putty
- Paste
- Strips
- Injectables
- Powder
- Gel

Ideal bone graft properties include (1) ability to serve the intended primary purpose (structural vs filling voids); (2) absent immunogenicity; (3) cost-effectiveness; (4) indefinite storage capability; (5) easy handling properties; (6) rapid incorporation; (7) stable fixation capability; and (8) osteoconductive (scaffold), osteoinductive (signal), and osteogenic (cells) properties. Osteoconductive properties allow the graft to serve as a scaffold or lattice-work for new bone formation. Graft incorporation is biologically complex, but it generally occurs by creeping substitution. Bone grafts with osteoinductive properties can direct the host's mesenchymal stem cells (pluripotential cells) into the host-graft interface to form bone. Host mesenchymal cells can be signaled to differentiate into osteoblasts. Finally, osteogenic grafts can synthesize new bone from cells within the graft or the host. Various products are available that incorporate several of these qualities.

BONE GRAFT PROCESSING AND STERILIZATION

Allograft processing and sterilization techniques may dramatically alter its properties and affect its quality and safety. Allograft tissues are regulated by the US Food and Drug Administration (FDA) and the American Association of Tissue Banks (AATB). It is important that foot and ankle surgeons are aware that AATB accreditation is not mandated by law. Therefore, it is recommended that surgeons use allografts from accredited AATB sources and know their bone banks' specific processing techniques.

Guidelines on appropriate and recommended procurement, sterilization, and storage techniques are available through the *Standards for Tissue Banking* manual, which is updated frequently by the AATB.[2] Eligibility of donors is determined by a series of standardized questionnaires, tests, physical examinations, medical record reviews, autopsy reports (if performed), and, of course, consent. Final approval for graft donation is determined by a licensed physician. Donors of musculoskeletal tissues are automatically ineligible if there was toxic substance exposure, significant bone disease, or autoimmune disease identification. Blood tests are used primarily for infectious disease screening. To decrease the amount of time it takes to detect viruses, nucleic acid testing (NAT) for human immunodeficiency virus (HIV) and hepatitis C virus (HCV) was initiated by the AATB in 2005.[3] Donors must test negative for antibodies to HIV, HCV, hepatitis B virus (HBV) surface antigen, total antibody to hepatitis B core antigen, antibodies to human T-lymphotropic virus (HTLV), and syphilis.[2]

Once a donor is identified and considered eligible, the procurement, timing, handling, and storage of the tissue must follow strict AATB guidelines. Aseptic techniques are standardized and implemented for all accredited AATB tissue banks. The tissue must be removed from a donor within 24 hours of asystole, if the body was cooled, or within 15 hours of death, if the body was not cooled (90% or more tissues are from hospitals). Following removal, the tissues are cultured. Once the cultures are negative, the musculoskeletal tissue processing is conducted in a sterile and climate-controlled environment.[2]

Secondary sterilization is then used with the intention of eliminating all possibility of infection from false positive cultures or from handling. This sterilization process must be effective in eradicating any possible bacteria, fungus, or virus, although still attempting to maintain the biologic and mechanical properties of the tissue. No technique currently exists that completely meets these requirements. Although ethylene oxide was previously a popular sterilization technique, most tissue banks have discontinued or minimized its use, because increased graft failure and chronic synovitis have been attributed to ethylene oxide.[4,5] If tissue banks use ethylene oxide as a secondary sterilization method, the AATB requires that the ethylene oxide and its breakdown products must be reduced below a specified level.[2] Gamma irradiation is another popular method of secondary sterilization. The highest known dose that does not significantly alter the biomechanical graft properties is 2.5 mrad. Most centers use a 2.5 mrad dose currently. Many studies have demonstrated that this dose is effective in eliminating bacterial surface contamination, but doses higher than 3 mrad are required to kill viruses.[4,5] Therefore, many additional proprietary techniques and even additional antibiotic soaks are usually implemented to augment irradiation.[4,5]

Companies are in constant search of the most complete secondary sterilization process, which is why there are many combinations and variations in techniques. Some of the newer sterilization techniques include BioCleanse (Regeneration Technologies, Gainesville, FL, USA), Allowash formula (LifeNet, Virginia Beach, VA, USA), and the Clearant Process (Clearant, Los Angeles, CA, USA). The sterilization process may use some form of irradiation along with a combination of chemical liquid sterilants, antibiotics, ultrasound, low-temperature or freezing techniques, and centrifugation.[6–9] Although in-house testing is performed and methods are FDA approved, peer-reviewed comparative literature and outcomes-based research is lacking on how proprietary processes affect bone graft properties, while still ensuring the maximum sterilization and safety.

Spread of disease or infection from musculoskeletal donor graft to host is considered to be of low risk by the Centers for Disease Control and Prevention and AATB. Potential pathogens in donor graft tissue may include (1) viruses (primarily HIV-1,-2; HCV; HBV; HTLV-1,-2); (2) bacteria (isolated examples in the literature include *Clostridium* species, *Staphylococcus aureus*, β-hemolytic streptococci, Enterobacteriaceae, *Pseudomonas* species, and *Enterococci*); (3) yeast; (4) mold and fungi; and (5) transmissible spongiform encephalopathies.[1,10,11] The risk of disease transmission depends on the type of allograft. Fresh and fresh-frozen allografts are considered to have a higher risk than others. Demineralized and freeze-dried allografts have had no disease transmission reports in the last 30 years, with the probability of HIV transmission estimated to be 1 in 2.8 billion.[10] This is attributed to the freeze-drying and demineralization processes and to the ability to delay processing for additional testing, without compromise in graft properties. The estimated risk of contracting HIV from other musculoskeletal allografts is believed to be 1 in 1.6 million.[4,5] Disease transmission for HCV and other viruses is unknown but is also believed to be rare.[12–17] The risk of HCV transmission has decreased even further because of the AATB's NAT requirements, which entail testing for the actual virus as opposed to antibodies to the virus.[3,17]

ALLOGRAFTS

Allografts are one of the most common alternative bone graft types used in reconstructive foot and ankle surgery. Allograft may be fresh, frozen or fresh-frozen, freeze-dried (lyophilized), or demineralized (decalcified).

Fresh Allografts

Osteochondral fresh allografts contain intact hyaline cartilage, with living chondrocytes, and a thin shell of cancellous bone that is kept intact because it is necessary for fixation. Therefore, they contain osteogenic, osteoinductive, and osteoconductive properties. Disadvantages include logistic and procurement limitations, increased immunogenicity and disease transmission possibilities, cost, and increased surgical technical demands, resulting in mixed outcomes. Fresh allograft use has been reported in the ankle, knee, and hip.[18–28]

After a rigorous screening and selection process (approved by the AATB), harvested fresh cadaveric allografts (donors <45 years old) are slowly cooled and stored in cell media at 4°C. According to the AATB, specimens can be stored in this manner for up to 6 weeks, but transplantation timing may influence outcomes.[29] Studies have found that chondrocyte viability, density, and metabolic activity significantly decrease after 14 days in storage ($P<.01$), whereas glycosaminoglycans and cartilage matrix properties remain preserved.[30] Safety testing, for a minimum of 14 days, is now required before release of fresh allografts because of AATB restrictions.[1,2,29] It is postulated that earlier studies may have shown more favorable outcomes because of average time from death to transplantation being less than 1 week; this time is now required to be at least 2 weeks.[23,24]

The graft size must also be precisely matched. Measurements from anteroposterior and lateral radiographs have been traditionally used for size matching; however, computer-assisted 3-dimensional programs, using CT reconstructions, may improve future allograft size selection.[31]

Fresh osteochondral allografts do not currently require tissue or blood-type matching between host and cadaver donors. It is thought that the matrix surrounding the living chondrocytes protects graft rejection by host cells.[32,33] Immunogenic responses are measured in patients by serum anti-HLA (human leukocyte antigen) antibodies, preoperatively, and 6 months postoperatively. In the largest, most recent series, 91% of the patients tested positive for HLA antibodies at 6 months. Anecdotal reports express the thought that allograft irrigation before transplantation may decrease the chance of graft rejection, because there may be fewer bone marrow elements.[19] Animal models further support the possibility of increased immunogenicity in mismatched specimens.[34,35]

Fresh osteochondral ankle replacement outcomes have been mixed. Overall, there are only case series available in the literature, with survival ranging from 31% to 92% at 2 to 12 years.[18–22] Reported modes of graft failure include graft fracture, graft collapse, loss of joint space, deep infection, nonunion, and malunion. To preserve cell viability, fresh allografts cannot be rigorously disinfected and sterilized in the same manner as other allografts. Despite concerns, rates of infection are reportedly low. Use of cutting jigs and external fixation assistance may decrease intraoperative technical errors. Although difficult to interpret because of small sample size and limited follow-up, it seems that host factors (BMI, malalignment, and age) may influence results.[20] Revision surgery from graft failure may require repeat transplantation, total ankle replacement, and arthrodesis, often with freeze-dried bone block or bulk allograft due to bone loss.[18–22]

Fresh-frozen Allografts

The main purpose of freezing fresh-frozen allograft is to reduce immunogenicity, increase shelf-life, and provide a more practical option than fresh allografts. It is performed in such a way as to preserve osteoconductive and osteoinductive properties and strength. Fresh-frozen allograft may be used when a partial or complete joint surface is being replaced or when a structural graft is required. Graft size must be matched, if used for partial or complete joint replacement or for whole or massive bone transplantation. Frozen grafts must be thawed intraoperatively and do not require rehydration.[2,36,37]

Frozen allograft may undergo conventional freezing ($-15°C$ to $-30°C$), deep freezing ($-60°C$ to $-80°C$), or freezing with liquid nitrogen ($-160°C$ to $-180°C$).[38] Most grafts are frozen to $-70°C$ to $-80°C$ and this temperature must stay within AATB ranges during transportation and storage.[39] Deep freezing may weaken the bone; it is thought that the graft maintains approximately 70% of normal bone strength. After the bone graft is frozen, it is sterilized.[40] Shelf-life varies anywhere from 1 to 10 years, depending on processing techniques. Each bone bank has unique guidelines, and only bone banks accredited by the AATB should be used.[1,36]

The degree of osteoinductive properties depends significantly on the fresh-frozen allograft processing and storage characteristics. If frozen too quickly or stored at improper temperatures, the graft may become completely acellular. Cryopreservation is used to freeze bone in a controlled manner so that water crystals do not damage viable cells, and biologically mediated termination, such as apoptosis, will not occur.[41] Lower temperatures have been found to render cells nonviable in animal models.[39,41,42]

Whole fresh-frozen bone replacement, in cases of massive bone loss due to tumors, has been reported. Whole calcaneal replacement has been successful in 2 cases of bone tumors (chondrosarcoma and giant cell tumor) with 32 and 9 years of follow-up. In both cases, the fresh-frozen calcaneus was fused to the talus and cuboid.[43] In another case report, after resection of a first metatarsal for a giant cell tumor, whole first metatarsal fresh-frozen allograft successfully fused to the proximal phalanx and medical cuneiform.[44]

Case reports for partial ankle joint replacement either for bone tumors, trauma, or select osteochondral defects have also been successful. Although early reports are encouraging, long term viability of partial joint replacement with fresh-frozen allograft is not available.[45–49] Finally, fresh-frozen allograft from femoral head allografts have been successfully used for numerous foot and ankle procedures.[50–52] The investigators have used femoral head allografts, in collaboration with Philip Basile, DPM, for Charcot neuroarthropathy deformity involving the talus (**Fig. 1**A, B).

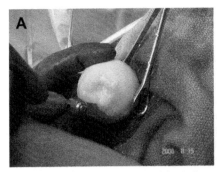
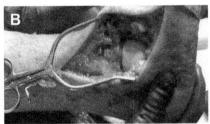

Fig.1. (*A*) Example of femoral head fresh frozen allograft. (*B*) To prevent the development of a calcaneal gait following removal of the talus, a femoral head allograft is used for deformity correction and tibiocalcaneal arthrodesis.

Freeze-dried (Lyophilized) Allografts

Freeze-dried allografts are the most common type of allograft currently used in foot and ankle surgery. After the allograft is frozen, it is lyophilized: it undergoes a dehydration process whereby water is removed under vacuum pressure. This process kills all viable cells, inactivates viral agents, and alters bone structure. Freeze-dried allograft advantages include its osteoconductive properties, its low antigenic potential, its ability to be stored at room temperature, its indefinite shelf life, and its lower cost compared with fresh and frozen alternatives. It cannot be used in massive tumor resection replacement because of reduced mechanical strength. Only 30% of normal bone strength is retained after processing and sterilization procedures. In addition, the surgeon must follow rehydration guidelines to avoid further increasing the brittleness of the bone graft.[1,2,53]

Freeze-dried allografts have been reported throughout the literature. They may be used for filling in voids (**Fig. 2**) or for structural purposes (**Fig. 3**A, B), depending on their form.[54] Freeze-dried allograft is commonly used in foot and ankle surgery to augment or assist in deformity correction for primary or revision ankle, rearfoot and midfoot arthrodeses, and osteotomies.[55–59] Allograft wedging can augment the

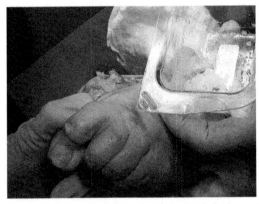

Fig. 2. Croutons are blocks of cancellous freeze-dried allograft that can be morselized or mixed with other bone grafts and is useful for filling in bony voids.

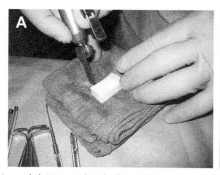
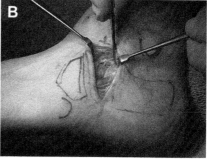

Fig. 3. (*A*) Freeze-dried allograft can be shaped and used to correct various foot and ankle deformities. (*B*) Example of allograft in use for pes plano valgus deformity correction.

correction one can achieve in pes plano valgus, pes cavus, and Charcot reconstructions. A small randomized trial that compared autogenous and tricortical iliac crest allograft, for lateral column lengthening in adult-acquired flatfoot, found that all patients achieved bony union by 12 weeks, regardless of graft type.[60]

Demineralized (Decalcified) Allograft

Demineralized allograft is essentially morselized allograft that has been sieved to specific particulate sizes. Hydrochloric acid demineralizes the bone matrix and extracts acid-soluble proteins. After successive washings, millings, and sterilization, it can be freeze-dried to allow storage at room temperatures. What remains is demineralized bone matrix (DBM), growth factors, collagen, proteoglycans, and bone morphogenic proteins (BMP). DBM has osteoconductive properties but no structural capabilities. Osteoinductive properties may be enhanced because of the presence of BMPs and numerous growth factors.

The type of carrier determines the form of DBM. Carriers include glycerol, gelatin, and calcium sulfate powder. DBM is available in putty, paste, gel, sheets, plugs, powder, and many other forms (**Fig. 4**). DBM is often combined with grafts that contain structural support but have few osteoinductive properties. It can be combined with

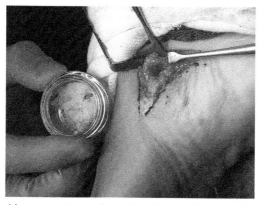

Fig. 4. Demineralized bone matrix may be packed into voids or combined with other types of bone graft.

autograft and various allografts to increase graft volume. Powder forms have been mixed with antibiotic.[61–63]

XENOGRAFTS

Until recently, xenograft implantation was avoided in foot and ankle surgery because of concerns about antigenicity and graft rejection. Advances in processing and sterilization techniques have now significantly reduced immunogenicity and permitted a new emergence in xenograft usage. Xenografts can provide structural support and osteoconduction; however, osteoinduction and osteogenesis are not possible.

Cancello-Pure (Wright Medical Technology, Arlington, TN, USA) is a bovine xenograft which comes from a US Department of Agriculture (USDA) certified, closed, organic herd. Extensive records are kept for this closed herd and no cases of bovine spongiform encephalopathy have ever been identified. Cancello-Pure uses Bio-Cleanse for its tissue sterilization process. BioCleanse is an FDA validated process that kills bacteria, fungal spores, and viruses, by combining proprietary techniques using stringent chemical liquid sterilants and irradiation. More than 300,000 allografts have been implanted using BioCleanse and there have been no reports of infection to date.[6,7] One of the greatest advantages of Cancello-Pure is reduced operating room time for common procedures, such as both Evans and Cotton opening-wedge osteotomies. This is because it is supplied in machined cortico-cancellous wedges that can be sized precisely using an innovative cutting jig (**Fig. 5**A–C). Cancello-Pure is also stored at room temperature and does not require rehydration.[64] Studies are needed

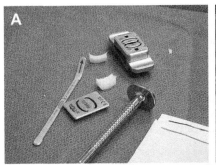
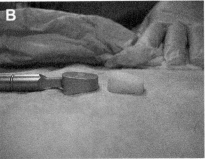
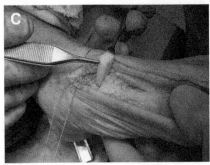

Fig. 5. (*A*) This cutting jig can cut precise wedges for both Evans and Cotton opening wedge osteotomies for pes plano valgus correction. (*B*) Xenograft allograft has been cut to the same size as the sizer used for pes plano valgus correction. (*C*) Xenograft allograft for Cotton opening wedge osteotomy.

to further determine its long-term viability, incorporation rate, biomechanical properties, and antigenicity.

Other xenografts may become available in the future. Healos (DePuy Spine, Raynham, MA, USA) is a bovine cross-linked collagen matrix that is coated with hydroxyapatite (HA) and comes in sponge-like strips. Feasibility studies have been performed comparing Healos (combined with autogenous bone marrow) with autogenous graft in lumbar spinal fusion, with favorable preliminary results.[65,66]

Collagraft (Zimmer Corporation, Warsaw, IN, USA) is a bovine collagen combined with HA (65%) and tricalcium phosphate (35%). When combined with bone marrow and internal or external fixation, Collagraft may be used for traumatic deficits or acute fractures in long bones.[67–72] Colloss E (Ossacur AG, Oberstenfeld, Germany) is a protein (mainly type I collagen) extracted from cortical diaphyseal equine long bones via lyophilization. Suitable carriers are still under investigation.[73,74] Both Collagraft and Colloss E are considered to have osteoinductive properties.[67,75]

SYNTHETIC BONE GRAFTS

Synthetic bone grafts are nonosseous artificial materials used as bone graft substitutes. The ideal synthetic bone graft should be biocompatible and have maximal osseointegration capabilities, osteoconduction, and a similar modulus of elasticity to the replaced bone. Unless combined with other products, synthetic bone grafts do not possess osteoinductive or osteogenic properties. Synthetic bone grafts do not carry a risk of disease transmission and can be formed in any desired shape or size. Synthetic bone grafts may be broadly categorized into calcium and silicon.[76]

Calcium Synthetic Bone Grafts

Calcium synthetic bone grafts may be broadly categorized as calcium sulfate or calcium phosphate. Calcium is versatile, being available in many different forms. These forms include powders, pellets, pastes, granules, blocks, ceramics, marine coral, and cements. Porosity varies considerably between products, with more porous materials undergoing more rapid degradation than denser forms. Most synthetic bone grafts have few or no structural properties due to brittle characteristics and are therefore primarily used for filling voids and to expand other grafts.

Calcium sulfate

Calcium sulfate ("Plaster of Paris", $CaSO_4$) has been used since the 1800s. It undergoes rapid dissolution within 5 to 7 weeks. It can be mixed with antibiotics and used for osteomyelitis. Its reported advantage over antibiotic-impregnated cement beads is that a second operation is not required to remove the substance. However, it is possible for serous drainage to develop, which is attributed to its rapid resorption rate. One commercially available form is Osteoset (Wright Medical Technology, Arlington, TN, USA), which is impregnated with tobramycin. Cerament Bone Void Filler (Bonesupport AB, Lund, Sweden) is another form but is a combination of calcium sulfate (60%) and HA (40%). Cerament is an injectable ceramic bone substitute in which the HA provides an osteoconductive matrix and may be applied to enhance implant integration.[77]

Calcium phosphates

There are several calcium phosphate ($CaPO_4$) varieties that are commercially available, including beta tricalcium phosphate (βTCP), synthetic HA, coralline HA, and calcium phosphate cements. Synthetic HA may be divided into ceramic or nonceramic forms. Ceramic is created by heating (sintering) HA crystals to form a larger crystalline structure. Coralline HA originates from marine coral (*Porites* and *Goniopora* species) and its processing and sterilization techniques convert it into calcium phosphate.

In general, calcium phosphate materials are more resistant to compressive loads but are brittle and may fracture under shock load, shear, and tension stresses. Their use in weight-bearing applications necessitates protective fixation until bony ingrowth has occurred. They are considered biocompatible and have osteoconductive properties. βTCP is the most porous and may undergo dissolution within 6 to 18 months. Conversely, ceramic HA forms are resistant to degradation, only undergoing 1% to 2% resorption per year.[76,78]

In recent years, combinations of calcium sulfate and calcium phosphate have been implemented to try and capture the major advantages of each material. One example with which the investigators have had experience is Pro-Dense (Wright Medical Technology, Arlington, TN, USA). Pro-Dense is an injectable paste that basically consists of three-fourths $CaSO_4$ (more rapid resorption) and one-fourth $CaPO_4$ (slower resorption). It is hypothesized that this composite is more biocompatible than pure $CaSO_4$, therefore decreasing risk of serous drainage postoperatively. Its matrix consists of both $CaSO_4$ and dicalcium phosphate dehydrate, which is thought to improve osteoconductive capabilities. After the $CaSO_4$ resorbs (approximately 6 weeks), there is still a residual porous matrix from the dicalcium phosphate dehydrate. βTCP granules are embedded within this matrix and are slowly replaced by bone.[79,80]

Animal studies have shown that this $CaSO_4/CaPO_4$ composite results in greater bone density in the replaced bone compared with $CaSO_4$ pellets alone ($P = .025$) and normal bone ($P = .008$). At 13 weeks and 26 weeks, the $CaSO_4/CaPO_4$ composite specimens demonstrated greater strength and compressive stress compared with $CaSO_4$ and normal bone ($P<.05$). In addition, the modulus of elasticity of the replaced bone was similar between the $CaSO_4/CaPO_4$ composite and normal bone at 13 and 26 weeks. Investigators did still find a small amount of $CaSO_4/CaPO_4$ composite at 26 weeks.[79] Clinically, this $CaSO_4/CaPO_4$ composite can be used to fill voids and augment hardware (**Fig. 6A–I**).[79,80] Additional studies are needed to further understand long-term viability and outcomes.

Silicon Synthetic Bone Grafts

Bioactive glasses and glass ionomers are silicon-based synthetic bone grafts. They have the ability to bond to bone by chemical processes and therefore exchange ions with the host bone. Because they are difficult to fixate and can fracture, they are primarily indicated as void fillers and bone graft expanders. Currently, they have few advantages over other materials. Bioactive ceramics were created to have increased strength, but they are still prone to fractures. Furthermore, bioactive glasses and ceramics have a higher modulus of elasticity than cortical bone. Glass ionomers are a nonabsorbable graft and therefore cannot become incorporated. They have been used as a sealant in dentistry and in skull and maxillofacial reconstruction.[76]

FACTOR- AND CELL-BASED BONE GRAFTS

BMPs are proteins found within bone that stimulate mesenchymal cells to differentiate into osteoblasts (osteoinductive properties). More than 15 BMPs have been identified to play a role in bone formation; however, only 3 have the capability of producing bone in ectopic locations: BMP-2, BMP-4, and BMP-7. Although only a tiny amount of BMP can be extracted from DBM, recombinant therapy is used for more efficient production. The 2 recombinant BMPs available commercially are rhBMP-2 (Infuse, Medtronic Sofamor Danek, Memphis, TN, USA) and rhBMP-7 osteogenic protein 1 (OP-1,

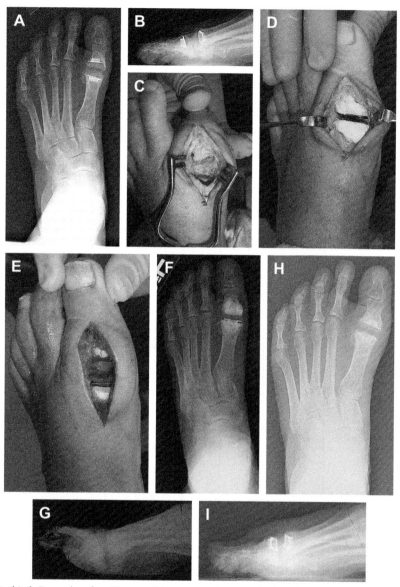

Fig. 6. (*A–I*) Example of a 54-year-old woman who required replacement of a total first metacarpophalangeal joint silicone implant. Pro-Dense injectable bone graft was used to prevent implant subsidence and to assist in proper positioning of the replacement implant because of excessive bone loss. (*A, B*) Preoperative radiographs demonstrating bony over-growth and severe implant subsidence. (*C*) A large deficit was present after removal of the failed implant and resection of pathologic tissue. (*D*) Bone graft paste was injected into the bony deficits and molded into shape for the metal grommets. (*E*) Insertion of a new total-hinged silicone implant. (*F, G*) Note the radiopaque bone graft substitute surrounding the implant postoperatively. (*H, I*) After 12 weeks, radiographs demonstrate that most of the bone graft substitute has been replaced. (*Courtesy of* Adam Landsman, DPM, PhD, Boston, MA.)

Table 2
Overview of alternative bone graft substitute properties[a]

Bone Graft Substitute Type	Requires Freezing or Refrigeration	Shelf Life	Antigenic Potential	Osteoconduction	Osteoinduction	Osteogenesis	Structural Support
Fresh allograft	Yes (≈4°C)	<6weeks	+++	+++	+++	±	+++
Fresh-frozen allograft	Yes (−70°C to −80°C is common)	1–5 years	++	+++	+	−	+++
Freeze-dried allograft	No (room temperature)	Indefinite	+	+++	±	−	++
Demineralized allograft	No (room temperature)	Indefinite	+	++	++	−	−
Xenograft	No (room temperature)	Indefinite	+	+++	−	−	+++
Synthetic bone graft	No (room temperature)	Indefinite	−	+++	−	−	±

[a] These are approximations that also depend on the shape and quantity of bone graft; refer to AATB and bone banking guidelines for the most current information.

Stryker Biotech, Hopkinton, MA, USA). Due to promising results for factor- and cell-based bone grafts, separate articles in this issue are dedicated to these important topics.

SUMMARY

The choice in bone graft can be overwhelming for the reconstructive foot and ankle surgeon. This article aims to provide important information regarding bone allografts, practical applications, and a classification for grouping new products as they become available. **Table 2** also summarizes the properties of each type of allograft as a rapid reference. Innovation and advances in reconstructive foot and ankle surgery have been coupled with an increase in the use of osseous allograft. Future studies are needed to further understand the outcomes and limitations of the different types of allograft and their processing procedures.

REFERENCES

1. American Association of Tissue Banks. Available at: http://www.aatb.org. Accessed February 01, 2009.
2. Standards for Tissue Banking 2006. Available at: http://www.aatb.org. Accessed February 01, 2009.
3. Rigney PR. Implementation of nucleic acid testing (NAT) 2004. Available at: http://www.aatb.org. Accessed March 25, 2009.
4. Caldwell PE III, Shelton WR. Indications for allografts. Orthop Clin North Am 2005; 36(4):459–67.
5. Rihn JA, Harner CD. The use of musculoskeletal allograft tissue in knee surgery. Arthroscopy 2003;19(Suppl 1):51–66.
6. Regeneration Technologies I. The BioCleanse process 2006. Available at: http://www.rtix.com/BiocleanseProcess.aspx. Accessed March 30, 2009.
7. Assessment of the antigenic response of sheep recipients following implantation of BioCleanse treated bovine bone, untreated bovine bone and untreated allograft bone 2007. Available at: http://www.wmt.com/Downloads/SO045-207%20CancelloPure%20WP.pdf. Accessed March 25, 2009.
8. Wolfinbarger L. Ensuring safety in tissue transplantation: the sterilization of allografts 2004. Available at: http://www.purgo.co.kr/data/_24172%20LifeNet%20Sterilization%20paper.pdf. Accessed March 26, 2009.
9. Clearant I. Bone allograft. The clearant process. Available at: http://www.clearant.com/bone.html. Accessed March 26, 2009.
10. Center for Biologics Evaluation and Research (CBER): tissues 2008. Available at: http://www.fda.gov/cber/tiss.htm. Accessed March 26, 2009.
11. Patel R, Trampuz A. Infections transmitted through musculoskeletal-tissue allografts. N Engl J Med 2004;350(25):2544–6.
12. Joyce MJ. Safety and FDA regulations for musculoskeletal allografts: perspective of an orthopaedic surgeon. Clin Orthop Relat Res 2005;435:22–30.
13. Mroz TE, Joyce MJ, Steinmetz MP, et al. Musculoskeletal allograft risks and recalls in the United States. J Am Acad Orthop Surg 2008;16(10):559–65.
14. Mroz TE, Joyce MJ, Lieberman IH, et al. The use of allograft bone in spine surgery: is it safe? Spine J 2009;9(4):303–8.
15. McAllister DR, Joyce MJ, Mann BJ, et al. Allograft update: the current status of tissue regulation, procurement, processing, and sterilization. Am J Sports Med 2007;35(12):2148–58.

16. Tomford WW. Transmission of disease through transplantation of musculoskeletal allografts. J Bone Joint Surg Am 1995;77(11):1742–54.

17. Tugwell BD, Patel PR, Williams IT, et al. Transmission of hepatitis C virus to several organ and tissue recipients from an antibody-negative donor. Ann Intern Med 2005;143(9):648–54.

18. Gross AE, Agnidis Z, Hutchison CR. Osteochondral defects of the talus treated with fresh osteochondral allograft transplantation. Foot Ankle Int 2001;22(5): 385–91.

19. Meehan R, McFarlin S, Bugbee W, et al. Fresh ankle osteochondral allograft transplantation for tibiotalar joint arthritis. Foot Ankle Int 2005;26(10):793–802.

20. Jeng CL, Kadakia A, White KL, et al. Fresh osteochondral total ankle allograft transplantation for the treatment of ankle arthritis. Foot Ankle Int 2008;29(6): 554–60.

21. Tontz WL Jr, Bugbee WD, Brage ME. Use of allografts in the management of ankle arthritis. Foot Ankle Clin 2003;8(2):361–73, xi.

22. Kim CW, Jamali A, Tontz W Jr, et al. Treatment of post-traumatic ankle arthrosis with bipolar tibiotalar osteochondral shell allografts. Foot Ankle Int 2002;23(12): 1091–102.

23. Meyers MH. Resurfacing of the femoral head with fresh osteochondral allografts. Long-term results. Clin Orthop Relat Res 1985;197:111–4.

24. Meyers MH, Akeson W, Convery FR. Resurfacing of the knee with fresh osteochondral allograft. J Bone Joint Surg Am 1989;71(5):704–13.

25. McGoveran BM, Pritzker KP, Shasha N, et al. Long-term chondrocyte viability in a fresh osteochondral allograft. J Knee Surg 2002;15(2):97–100.

26. Mahomed MN, Beaver RJ, Gross AE. The long-term success of fresh, small fragment osteochondral allografts used for intraarticular post-traumatic defects in the knee joint. Orthopedics 1992;15(10):1191–9.

27. Ghazavi MT, Pritzker KP, Davis AM, et al. Fresh osteochondral allografts for post-traumatic osteochondral defects of the knee. J Bone Joint Surg Br 1997;79(6): 1008–13.

28. Shasha N, Krywulak S, Backstein D, et al. Long-term follow-up of fresh tibial osteochondral allografts for failed tibial plateau fractures. J Bone Joint Surg Am 2003;85(Suppl 2):33–9.

29. Farr J. Current concepts: fresh osteochondral shell allografts 2001. Available at: http://www.aatb.org/files/2001Abstract4.pdf. Accessed February 01, 2009.

30. Williams SK, Amiel D, Ball ST, et al. Prolonged storage effects on the articular cartilage of fresh human osteochondral allografts. J Bone Joint Surg Am 2003; 85(11):2111–20.

31. Aponte-Tinao L, Ritacco L, Farfalli G, et al. Computer-assisted 3D preoperative planning for allograft selection in orthopedic reconstructions. 2008. Available at: http://www.aatb.org/files/s608annual.pdf. Accessed January 12, 2009.

32. Langer F, Czitrom A, Pritzker KP, et al. The immunogenicity of fresh and frozen allogeneic bone. J Bone Joint Surg Am 1975;57(2):216–20.

33. Langer F, Gross AE. Immunogenicity of allograft articular cartilage. J Bone Joint Surg Am 1974;56(2):297–304.

34. Stevenson S, Dannucci GA, Sharkey NA, et al. The fate of articular cartilage after transplantation of fresh and cryopreserved tissue-antigen-matched and mismatched osteochondral allografts in dogs. J Bone Joint Surg Am 1989;71(9): 1297–307.

35. Stevenson S, Li XQ, Martin B. The fate of cancellous and cortical bone after transplantation of fresh and frozen tissue-antigen-matched and

mismatched osteochondral allografts in dogs. J Bone Joint Surg Am 1991; 73(8):1143–56.

36. Andrade MG, Sa CN, Marchionni AM, et al. Effects of freezing on bone histological morphology. Cell Tissue Bank 2008;9(4):279–87.

37. Steps in the tissue donation process. Available at: http://www.aatb.org/files/ stepsinthetissuedonationprocess.pdf. Accessed February 01, 2009.

38. Benzel E, Leon SP. Enhancing cervical spine fusion. 2001. Available at: http:// www.medscape.com/viewprogram/161_pnt. Accessed February 01, 2009.

39. Laitinen M, Kivikari R, Hirn M. Lipid oxidation may reduce the quality of a fresh-frozen bone allograft. Is the approved storage temperature too high? Acta Orthop 2006;77(3):418–21.

40. Eagle MJ, Rooney P, Lomas R, et al. Validation of radiation dose received by frozen unprocessed and processed bone during terminal sterilisation. Cell Tissue Bank 2005;6(3):221–30.

41. Simpson D, Kakarala G, Hampson K, et al. Viable cells survive in fresh frozen human bone allografts. Acta Orthop 2007;78(1):26–30.

42. Ohlendorf C, Tomford WW, Mankin HJ. Chondrocyte survival in cryopreserved osteochondral articular cartilage. J Orthop Res 1996;14(3):413–6.

43. Muscolo DL, Ayerza MA, Aponte-Tinao LA. Long-term results of allograft replacement after total calcanectomy. A report of two cases. J Bone Joint Surg Am 2000; 82(1):109–12.

44. Wang EH, Arbatin JJ. Allograft reconstruction of a large giant cell tumor of the first metatarsal: a case report. Foot Ankle Int 2008;29(1):97–100.

45. Schoenfeld AJ, Leeson MC, Grossman JP. Fresh-frozen osteochondral allograft reconstruction of a giant cell tumor of the talus. J Foot Ankle Surg 2007;46(3): 144–8.

46. Raikin SM. Stage VI: massive osteochondral defects of the talus. Foot Ankle Clin 2004;9(4):737–44, vi.

47. Thomas MI, Anderson JC, Hatch DJ, et al. Repair of an osteochondral tumor of the talus utilizing a fresh-frozen cadaveric graft. J Foot Ankle Surg 1997;36(5): 375–80 [discussion: 396].

48. Rubel IF, Carrer A. Fresh-frozen osteochondral allograft reconstruction of a severely fractured talus. A case report. J Bone Joint Surg Am 2005;87(3):625–9.

49. San-Julian M, Duart J, de Rada PD, et al. Limb salvage in Ewing's sarcoma of the distal lower extremity. Foot Ankle Int 2008;29(1):22–8.

50. Schuberth JM, Jennings MM. Reconstruction of the extruded talus with large allograft interfaces: a report of 3 cases. J Foot Ankle Surg 2008;47(5):476–82.

51. Garras DN, Santangelo JR, Wang DW, et al. Subtalar distraction arthrodesis using interpositional frozen structural allograft. Foot Ankle Int 2008;29(6):561–7.

52. Myerson MS, Neufeld SK, Uribe J. Fresh-frozen structural allografts in the foot and ankle. J Bone Joint Surg Am 2005;87(1):113–20.

53. Nather A. Biology and biomechanics healing of deep frozen and freeze-dried cortical bone allografts. 2002. Available at: http://www.aatb.org/files/ 2002Abstract69.pdf. Accessed February 01, 2009.

54. Rao S, McKellop H, Chao D, et al. Biomechanical comparison of bone graft used in anterior spinal reconstruction. Freeze-dried demineralized femoral segments versus fresh fibular segments and tricortical iliac blocks in autopsy specimens. Clin Orthop Relat Res 1993;289:131–5.

55. Campanacci DA, Scoccianti G, Beltrami G, et al. Ankle arthrodesis with bone graft after distal tibia resection for bone tumors. Foot Ankle Int 2008;29(10): 1031–7.

56. Carr CR, Hyatt GW. Clinical evaluation of freeze-dried bone grafts. J Bone Joint Surg Am 1955;37(3):549–66.

57. Mahan KT, Hillstrom HJ. Bone grafting in foot and ankle surgery. A review of 300 cases. J Am Podiatr Med Assoc 1998;88(3):109–18.

58. Templin D, Jones K, Weiner DS. The incorporation of allogeneic and autogenous bone graft in healing of lateral column lengthening of the calcaneus. J Foot Ankle Surg 2008;47(4):283–7.

59. Engh GA, Ammeen DJ. Use of structural allograft in revision total knee arthroplasty in knees with severe tibial bone loss. J Bone Joint Surg Am 2007;89(12):2640–7.

60. Dolan CM, Henning JA, Anderson JG, et al. Randomized prospective study comparing tri-cortical iliac crest autograft to allograft in the lateral column lengthening component for operative correction of adult acquired flatfoot deformity. Foot Ankle Int 2007;28(1):8–12.

61. Bibbo C, Patel DV. The effect of demineralized bone matrix-calcium sulfate with vancomycin on calcaneal fracture healing and infection rates: a prospective study. Foot Ankle Int 2006;27(7):487–93.

62. Pacaccio DJ, Stern SF. Demineralized bone matrix: basic science and clinical applications. Clin Podiatr Med Surg 2005;22(4):599–606, vii.

63. Park IH, Micic ID, Jeon IH. A study of 23 unicameral bone cysts of the calcaneus: open chip allogeneic bone graft versus percutaneous injection of bone powder with autogenous bone marrow. Foot Ankle Int 2008;29(2):164–70.

64. Cancello-pure wedges: alternative to cancellous allograft. 2008. Available at: http://www.wmt.com/footandankle/FA431-1107.asp. Accessed February 01, 2009.

65. Healos bone graft replacement. 2009. Available at: http://www.depuyspine.com/products/biologicssolutions/healos.asp. Accessed April 02, 2009.

66. Kitchel SH. A preliminary comparative study of radiographic results using mineralized collagen and bone marrow aspirate versus autologous bone in the same patients undergoing posterior lumbar interbody fusion with instrumented posterolateral lumbar fusion. Spine J 2006;6(4):405–11 [discussion: 411–2].

67. Collagraft: Zimmer foot and ankle solutions. Available at: http://www.zimmer.co.uk/web/enUS/pdf/product_brochures/Zimmer_Foot_and_Ankle_Brochure.pdf. Accessed April 02, 2009.

68. Kocialkowski A, Wallace WA, Prince HG. Clinical experience with a new artificial bone graft: preliminary results of a prospective study. Injury 1990;21(3):142–4.

69. Chapman MW, Bucholz R, Cornell C. Treatment of acute fractures with a collagen-calcium phosphate graft material. A randomized clinical trial. J Bone Joint Surg Am 1997;79(4):495–502.

70. Heijink A, Yaszemski MJ, Patel R, et al. Local antibiotic delivery with OsteoSet, DBX, and collagraft. Clin Orthop Relat Res 2006;451:29–33.

71. Leupold JA, Barfield WR, An YH, et al. A comparison of ProOsteon, DBX, and collagraft in a rabbit model. J Biomed Mater Res B Appl Biomater 2006;79(2):292–7.

72. Cornell CN, Lane JM, Chapman M, et al. Multicenter trial of collagraft as bone graft substitute. J Orthop Trauma 1991;5(1):1–8.

73. Boden SD. Evaluation of carriers of bone morphogenetic protein for spinal fusion. Spine 2001;26(8):850.

74. Lode A, Bernhardt A, Kroonen K, et al. Development of a mechanically stable support for the osteoinductive biomaterial COLLOSS E. J Tissue Eng Regen Med 2009;3(2):149–52.

75. Colloss E. Synthetic bone graft substitutes. Available at: http://www.ossacur. com/sites/colloss%20eng/colloss_europa_e.htm. Accessed February 01, 2009.
76. Moore WR, Graves SE, Bain GI. Synthetic bone graft substitutes. ANZ J Surg 2001;71(6):354–61.
77. Hatten H. The biomechanical and clinical efficacy of CERAMENT, a bi-phasic bone substitute for the treatment of vertebral compression fractures. J Vasc Interv Radiol 2009;20(2):S5.
78. Jarcho M. Calcium phosphate ceramics as hard tissue prosthetics. Clin Orthop Relat Res 1981;157:259–78.
79. Urban RM, Turner TM, Hall DJ, et al. Increased bone formation using a calcium sulfate and calcium phosphate composite graft. Clin Orthop Relat Res 2007; 459:110–7.
80. Panchbhavi VK, Vallurupalli S, Morris R, et al. The use of calcium sulfate and calcium phosphate composite graft to augment screw purchase in osteoporotic ankles. Foot Ankle Int 2008;29(6):593–600.

Bone Growth Stimulation for Foot and Ankle Nonunions

Crystal L. Ramanujam, DPM, Ronald Belczyk, DPM,
Thomas Zgonis, DPM, FACFAS*

KEYWORDS

• Revisional surgery • Bone growth stimulation
• Foot • Ankle • Nonunions

Bone healing requires a sequence of events to restore the integrity and biomechanical properties of the bone. Almost 6 million fractures occur annually in the United States, and 5% to 10% of these are reported to be complicated by nonunion and delayed union.[1] Although successful treatment of bony nonunions with bone growth stimulation can be found dating from the nineteenth century,[2,3] Fukada and Yasuda[4] first reported on the piezoelectricity of bone and the electrical stimulation of callus formation in the 1950s. Since then, considerable research has concentrated on the use of different methods of electromagnetism in bone healing, particularly on its effects in established nonunions.

The potential for delayed union or nonunion is increased in the presence of local and systemic risk factors. Local risk factors for delayed unions or nonunions include (and are not limited to) fracture site with poor blood supply, fracture comminution, bone gap, infection, and extensive soft tissue damage. Conditions such as smoking, diabetes mellitus, alcohol abuse, and older age are documented as systemic risk factors for nonunions.[5] Traditionally, treatment of delayed unions and nonunions has included open surgical fixation with autogenous bone grafting. The advantage of this method is that it provides osteoprogenitor cells and the necessary biologic components and scaffold for osteoinduction and osteoconduction. However, this method has limited options and is associated with donor site morbidity.[5] As a result, other mechanical, electrical, and chemical approaches have been developed, with electrical bone stimulation representing a $500 million market in the United States alone.[6,7]

Division of Podiatric Medicine and Surgery, Department of Orthopaedic Surgery, The University of Texas Health Science Center at San Antonio, San Antonio, TX, USA
* Corresponding author. Division of Podiatric Medicine and Surgery, Department of Orthopaedic Surgery, The University of Texas Health Science Center at San Antonio, San Antonio, TX.
E-mail address: zgonis@uthscsa.edu (T. Zgonis).

Clin Podiatr Med Surg 26 (2009) 607–618
doi:10.1016/j.cpm.2009.08.003
0891-8422/09/$ – see front matter © 2009 Elsevier Inc. All rights reserved.

Commonly, bone growth stimulation is used in the lower extremity for the following clinical scenarios: delayed union and nonunion of tibial fractures, ankle fractures, midfoot fractures, fifth metatarsal metaphyseal-diaphyseal junction fractures, and certain high-risk operations such as arthrodesis in the foot and ankle in patients with local or systemic risk factors for nonunion.

BIOLOGY AND PHYSIOLOGY OF BONE GROWTH STIMULATION

Healing response in bone cells requires unique cellular pathways to restore the normal form and function of the involved bone, including establishment of electric current or bioelectric potentials when the bone is stressed. This piezoelectric potential combined with transmembrane potentials generated by cellular metabolism in traumatized bone provides biophysical stimuli that favor the proper healing process.[8] In nonunions, these potentials within the tissue are in a disorganized, continuous "lag" phase.[9,10] Based on this premise, exogenous electrical potentials provided via electrical bone stimulators can enhance and amplify the physiologic bone healing response in the damaged tissues of nonunions.

On the cellular level, electrical stimulation has been shown to directly affect not only proliferation of osteoprogenitor cells from periosteal cells but also differentiation of osteoprogenitor cells to osteoblasts and finally to osteocytes by upregulation of local growth factors such as transforming growth factor-β1.[11,12] Molecular mechanisms of electrical stimulation-induced signal transduction have been described by Brighton and colleagues[13] which result in an increase in intracellular calcium, resulting in increased intracellular calmodulin and cell proliferation.

Mechanically induced bone formation requires nitric oxide and prostaglandin release, both of which have been shown to increase with exposure to low-intensity pulsed ultrasound (LIPUS).[14] Beneficial effects of these pulses include a positive impact on signal transduction, gene expression, blood flow, and tissue remodeling via increased collagen fiber formation and arrangement.[15] A molecular study by Hou and colleagues[16] demonstrated the signaling pathway in which ultrasound stimulates nuclear factor-κB activation and inducible nitric oxide synthase expression, which leads to nitric oxide production in preosteoblasts.

Historically, the definitions of delayed union and nonunion have been based on time from the onset of injury. The exact time frames are considered to be less important. Fracture healing is a dynamic, progressive process, and intervention is warranted within 3 to 5 months after injury if monthly radiographic studies do not show progression of fracture healing.[17] Nonunions of long bones are classically described by the Weber-Cech[18] classification as hypertrophic, atrophic, or normotrophic, according to their radiographic appearance. Electrical bone stimulation has been demonstrated to be the most effective method in the treatment of hypertrophic nonunions.[1]

TYPES OF BONE GROWTH STIMULATION DEVICES

The devices that are commercially available include, but are not limited to, the following: (1) direct current (DC), (2) capacitive coupling (CC), (3) pulsed electromagnetic field (PEMF), (4) combined electromagnetic field (CMF), and (5) LIPUS. All of these devices can be applied in conjunction with any method of stabilization or osteosynthesis (**Table 1**).

Direct Current

DC devices, first described by Paterson,[19] involve the generation of an electric current by a cathode and an anode, which are placed directly on the bone to be stimulated.

Table 1
Overview of current bone growth stimulation devices

Type of Bone Stimulation	Indications	Advantages/Disadvantages	Available Products
Direct current	Nonunions, congenital pseudoarthrosis	Advantages: increased compliance, direct current application, constant stimulation Disadvantages: need for second operation, local irritation, prominent hardware, pain	OsteoGen (EBI Medical Systems LP, Parsippany, NJ)
Capacitative coupling	Nonunions	Advantages: continuous, relatively noninvasive Disadvantages: long periods of use required, local discomfort from percutaneous placement of electrodes	Bioelectron Orthopak (EBI Medical Systems LP, Parsippany, NJ)
Pulsed electromagnetic field	Nonunions, congenital pseudoarthrosis, failed fusions	Advantages: noninvasive, can be used over cast Disadvantages: long periods of use required	EBI Bone Healing System (EBI Medical Systems LP, Parsippany, NJ) Physio-Stim Lite (Orthofix, Inc, McKinney, TX)
Combined magnetic field	Nonunions	Advantages: noninvasive, shorter periods of use Disadvantages: strict compliance	DonJoy OL1000 (Orthologic, Inc, Vista, CA)
Low-intensity pulsed ultrasound	Fresh fractures, nonunions	Advantages: noninvasive, short periods of use Disadvantages: strict compliance	Exogen (Smith & Nephew, Inc, Memphis, TN)

Although these devices allow weight bearing, 2 operations are needed to insert and remove the electrodes from the extremity if problems such as pain, infection, or prominent hardware occur. Advantages theoretically include increased compliance and constant stimulation of the nonunion site.

Only a few experiments demonstrating the possible efficacy of electrical stimulation on the healing of nonunions have been conducted on animals. Petersson and Johnell[20] have simulated nonunions in rabbit fibulae by placing a silicone spacer bilaterally in fresh fracture gaps. After 48 days, the spacers were removed, and DC was applied to 1 fibula and a sham device was applied to the contralateral fibula, serving as a control, for 62 days. Radiographic assessment showed that only 1 of the 6 rabbits developed overbridging callus at the nonunion site that was stimulated by DC, whereas none of the unstimulated fibulae showed bridging callus. Histologic analysis of the nonunions revealed only slightly more activity around the bony ends on the nonunions that were treated with DC.

Kleczynski[21] investigated the effect of DC in a fresh osteotomy model; fibular osteotomies in 12 rabbits were treated for 21 days with either DC therapy or placebo treatment. As in the Petersson study, no significant differences were observed in radiographic healing (as measured by the extent of periosteal and endosteal callus) and histologic healing reactions (as measured by osteoid formation).

A level IV case series by Brighton and colleagues[22] reported on 178 nonunions (including 90 tibial shafts, 13 medial malleoli, and 1 fibula) that were treated with a 12-week DC regimen followed by 12 weeks of cast immobilization, which resulted in bony union in 84% of all patients and in 74% of patients with a history of osteomyelitis.

In a similar level IV study, Kleczynski[21] found an 88% union rate for mainly tibial nonunions in a 34-patient series. The time to healing was notable, with a mean of more than 10 months. In contrast, Ahl and colleagues[23] found a substantially lower proportion (43%) of healed nonunions, and they attributed 7 of 13 failures to mobility of the nonunion.

Paterson and colleagues[24] presented a multicenter level IV case series of 84 patients, including 72 tibial nonunions treated by DC devices, resulting in bony union in 72 patients (86%) in an average of 16 weeks. These authors attributed the failures to improper placement of the cathode or too quick discontinuation of cast immobilization (**Table 2**).

Table 2 The effects of DC		
Study	Level of Evidence	Observations
Paterson et al, 1980[24]	IV	Series of 84 nonunions showed complete bony union in 86% with DC and cast immobilization on average of 16 wk
Brighton et al, 1981[22]	IV	Series of 178 nonunions demonstrated complete bony union in 84% with 12wk DC + 12 wk cast immobilization
Petersson et al, 1983[20]	I	Nonunion rabbit models revealed only slightly increased histologic activity at bony ends of those treated with DC
Kleczynski, 1988[21]	I	Fresh osteotomy rabbit model revealed no differences between DC vs placebo

Capacitative Coupling

In CC devices, electric fields are generated by 2 skin electrodes placed on opposite sides of the bone to be stimulated. The electrodes of these devices are placed percutaneously over the area of interest.[8] Similar to DC devices, weight bearing is possible with CC devices. Disadvantages include issues with compliance and pain from percutaneous placement of the electrodes.

Brighton and Pollack[25] first described outcomes of patients with nonunions treated by CC in a level IV study treating 22 nonunions, including 10 tibial fractures, for a mean of 25 weeks. Complete osseous union was noted in 17 patients (77%) after an average of 22.5 weeks. The only electrical stimulation-related complication noted was a local skin rash from the application of an electrode.

Scott and King[26] performed a level I prospective double-blind trial of 21 patients with femoral and tibial shaft nonunions; 10 patients received CC treatment and the remaining 11 received a sham bone stimulation device. Six patients in the treatment group achieved healing and none in the control group, which was a statistically significant result ($P<.004$).

A case series by Sarmiento and colleagues[27] provided a healing rate of 73% after CC treatment of tibial nonunions during 26 weeks (**Table 3**).

Pulsed Electromagnetic Fields (Inductive Coupling)

In PEMF, also known as inductive coupling, an external coil mounts an electromagnetic field not only between its cathode and anode but also in the direction of the nonunion.[25,28,29] PEMF is noninvasive but does not allow weight bearing. Response to treatment via this method is related to dose, frequency, amplitude, and duration of treatment; therefore, issues with compliance can be a major disadvantage.[5]

Ibiwoye and colleagues[30] created bilateral 6-mm osteotomies in rat fibulae, which were allowed to reach a nonunion state after 28 days, and then subjected them to a PEMF waveform for 3 h/d for 10 weeks. The study demonstrated a significant reduction in the amount of time-dependent bone volume loss in the distal fibular segments and a significantly smaller osteotomy gap in the limbs exposed to PEMF.

Several level IV studies on PEMF exist, with reported consolidation rates ranging from 64% to 90%. Because these studies are based on patient samples larger than those used in DC and CC studies, these values seem more valid than the union rates reported for CC and DC. In the largest of these series, Heckman and colleagues[31] reported that out of a total of 149 nonunions, including 94 tibial, only 96 nonunions (64%)

Table 3 The effects of CC		
Study	Level of Evidence	Observed Effects
Brighton & Pollack, 1985[25]	IV	Series of 22 nonunions showed complete osseous union in 77% treated with CC on average of 22.5 wk; 1 complication was local skin rash
Sarmiento et al, 1989[27]	IV	Tibial nonunions with CC showed 73% achieved healing in 26 wk
Scott and King, 1994[26]	I	21 femoral and tibial nonunions: 11 control and 10 with CC showed that 6 of 10 in study group achieved healing

progressed to union. The authors suggested the restriction of weight bearing, a possibly low compliance, and a lack of knowledge about PEMF devices as causes for the low overall healing rate.

In a level I multicenter prospective double-blind study of 45 patients with tibial delayed unions by Sharrard,[32] 12 weeks of PEMF for 20 patients compared with 12 weeks of sham treatment for 25 patients demonstrated a statistically significant difference ($P = .02$), with union achieved in 9 patients from the treatment group and in only 3 from the control group. In another large series, investigated by authors with more experience with PEMF, union was achieved in 87% of 127 patients.[33]

Fox and Smith[34] reported positive results in a case series applying PEMF to repair nonunions of metatarsals. In a small level IV case series involving 9 patients with delayed unions or nonunions of proximal fifth metatarsal fractures, Holmes[35] demonstrated mean healing time of 3 months for those treated with PEMF and non–weight bearing cast compared with mean healing time of 4.5 months for those treated with PEMF and weight bearing cast (**Table 4**).

Combined Electromagnetic Fields

Devices using CMFs use 2 external coiled-copper transducers to create 2 parallel low-energy magnetic fields. These devices appear to stimulate bone growth more quickly than the other types, can be used for shorter periods of time per day, and also require a smaller percentage of power.

Studies by Fitzsimmons and colleagues[36,37] have shown CMF to increase bone proliferation by mechanisms such as stimulating production of insulin-like growth factor and increasing calcium flux in bone cultures. A prospective, double-blind, placebo-controlled study by Linovitz and colleagues[38] demonstrated that CMF treatment of 30 min/d increases the probability of successful lumbar spine fusion.

In 1998, Hanft and colleagues[39] reported the first study to demonstrate the effects of CMF combined with immobilization in the treatment of Charcot neuroarthropathy.

Table 4 The effects of PEMF		
Study	Level of Evidence	Observed Effects
Bassett et al, 1981[33]	IV	Series of 127 patients showed osseous union in 87%; demonstrated that more experience with PEMF may lead to better results
Heckman et al, 1981[31]	IV	Large series of nonunions showed only 64% successful healing; suggested that restriction of weight bearing, low compliance, and lack of familiarity with device contributes to low healing rate
Sharrard, 1990[32]	I	45 patients with tibial delayed unions, 20 patients treated with PEMF compared with 25 in control group; 9 in study group achieved osseous union compared with only 3 in control group (statistically significant result)
Ibiwoye et al, 2004[30]	V	Rabbit model showed reduction in the amount of time-dependent bone volume loss in the distal fibular segments and a significantly smaller osteotomy gap in the limbs exposed to PEMF

These authors analyzed the time to radiographic consolidation in 31 subjects, 10 control subjects and 21 study subjects, with Charcot neuroarthropathy ranging from forefoot to ankle deformity. There was a statistically significant reduction in consolidation time, 23.8 weeks in the control group compared with 11 weeks in the study group.

Low-Intensity Pulsed Ultrasound

The LIPUS device is an external unit composed of a transducer that emits ultrasound waves through the skin and soft tissues to penetrate the bone at the site of interest. Currently, LIPUS is noninvasive and requires strict compliance. In contrast, recent experimental studies have proved the efficacy of a transosseous LIPUS application for enhancement and monitoring of the bone-healing process, in which miniature ultrasound transducers are surgically implanted into the fracture region.[40] LIPUS use has no known or reported complications. An additional advantage of this method over older electromagnetic stimulation is the requirement of much shorter treatment sessions, 20 min/d compared with several hours with the other devices (**Fig. 1**).

With the use of LIPUS in experimental osteotomy models using rabbit fibulae, Duarte[41] demonstrated an increase in bone callus formation. Pilla and colleagues[42] performed a placebo-controlled study of bilateral fibular osteotomies in rabbits, which demonstrated accelerated recovery of torsional strength and stiffness through application of LIPUS for 20 min/d. A study by Takikawa and colleagues[43] evaluated the effect of LIPUS on rat tibial nonunions, resulting in 50% of LIPUS-treated nonunions healing after 6 weeks compared with none of the tibial fractures in the control group. Xavier and Duarte[44] obtained a healing rate of 70% in 26 nonunions. In 1998, Strauss and Gonya[45] reported on the clinical use of low-intensity ultrasound for the treatment of Charcot arthropathy of the ankle. Since then, most studies have been performed to study the effect of LIPUS on healing of fresh fractures, many in a randomized controlled fashion. Heckman and colleagues[46] performed the first of this kind of study on fresh tibial fractures, which showed a 38% reduction in time to healing in the LIPUS treatment group compared with the control group (**Table 5**).

BONE GROWTH STIMULATION FOR FOOT AND ANKLE ARTHRODESIS

There is sufficient evidence in the literature supporting the use of bone growth stimulation as an adjunctive therapy for nonunions in high-risk patients. Cohen and colleagues[47] first reported on the successful use of a DC stimulator for treatment of a nonunion of the first metatarsal cuneiform joint, 8 months after attempted midfoot fusion for Charcot arthropathy. In a level IV study by Donley and Ward,[48] the authors reviewed the effect of DC stimulation for high-risk primary hindfoot fusions (ankle, subtalar, tibiotalocalcaneal, and tibiocalcaneal) in 13 patients. High-risk patients were defined as having a minimum of 2 major risk factors for nonunion, such as smoking, previous nonunion, previous infection, and osteonecrosis. Complete fusion with minimal complications was achieved in all but 1 patient. A similar level IV multicenter study by Saxena and colleagues[49] explored the use of DC stimulation in 26 high-risk patients undergoing 28 foot and ankle arthrodeses, with all patients having diabetes, elevated body mass index, previous failed arthrodeses, history of smoking or alcohol abuse, and/or chronic steroid use. Radiographic fusion occurred in 24 of the procedures at an average of 10.3 ± 4.0 weeks. The study showed that patients with 2 or more risk factors were more likely to require additional surgery for successful union.

Dhawan and colleagues[50] evaluated the use of PEMF on 64 patients undergoing triple or subtalar arthrodesis, including primary and revisional cases, in a level I

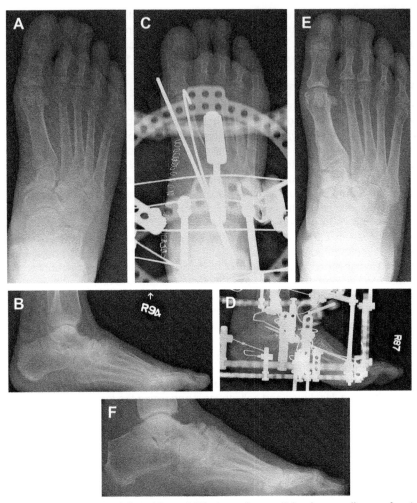

Fig. 1. An anteroposterior (A) and lateral (B) view of a medial column collapse of a right Charcot foot. Postoperative views (C, D) showing the medial column arthrodesis with the use of a multiplane circular fixation (C) and external bone growth stimulation (D). Radiographic views at 1-year follow-up, showing the medial column arthrodesis at the talonavicular-cuneiform joints (E, F).

prospective randomized clinical trial. Patients were divided into a control group and a PEMF group in which these patients used a PEMF device applied over a cast for 12 hours a day. The study analyzed 144 joints and showed that PEMF may accelerate the radiologic union rate of primary hindfoot arthrodesis.

There are few studies on the use of electrostimulation in specifically revisional arthrodesis. A level IV case series by Midis and Conti[51] used DC devices for revisional arthrodeses of aseptic ankle nonunions, with all 10 patients in the study achieving successful fusion at an average of 12.8 weeks. Saltzman and colleagues[52] found a relatively low success rate with PEMF in a level IV retrospective case series of 19 nonunion foot and ankle arthrodeses. In this study, only 26% achieved successful

Table 5
The effects of LIPUS

Study	Level of Evidence	Observed Effects
Duarte, 1983[41]	IV	Rabbit fibula osteotomy model showed increased bone callus with treatment by LIPUS
Xavier and Duarte, 1983[44]	IV	Observational study of 26 nonunions showed healing rate of 70% with LIPUS
Pilla et al, 1990[42]	I	LIPUS not only had an effect on the quantity of callus but also significantly increased the mechanical strength and stiffness of the callus
Heckman et al, 1994[46]	I	Study of fresh tibial fractures showed a significant (38%) reduction in time to healing in the LIPUS treatment group compared with that in the control group
Strauss and Gonya, 1998[45]	IV	Case study of LIPUS used in treatment of ankle Charcot arthropathy showed delay in progression of deformity
Takikawa et al, 2001[43]	I	Rat tibial nonunion fracture model showed 50% healing with LIPUS compared with none in the control group after 6 wk

union with their treatment protocol using PEMF, immobilization, and limited weight bearing.

The rising prevalence of diabetes and associated risk of Charcot arthropathy has prompted studies on the use of electrical bone stimulators specifically in this patient population undergoing arthrodesis.[53–55] In a level IV study of 10 Charcot patients, Hockenbury and colleagues[55] reviewed the results of arthrodeses (6 tibiotalocalcaneal, 2 pantalar, and 2 tibiocalcaneal) with concomitant use of an implantable bone growth stimulator. The authors found a fusion rate of 90% at an average of 3.7 months.

Jones and colleagues[56] reviewed a series of 13 patients with hindfoot nonunions that were treated with 10 subtalar and 3 triple revision arthrodeses accompanied by LIPUS. Coughlin and colleagues[57] provided the first level II prospective comparative study to evaluate LIPUS in primary subtalar arthrodesis patients. These authors found a 100% fusion rate in the 15 patients who received adjunctive ultrasound stimulation, with a statistically significant faster healing rate on plain radiographs and computed tomography scan compared with a similar cohort of patients who did not receive LIPUS therapy.

DISCUSSION

There is ample literature providing preclinical and observational findings suggesting the positive effects of adjunctive use of bone growth stimulation in nonunions of the foot and ankle. Significant attention has been paid to the application of bone stimulation in the treatment of long bone nonunion and foot and ankle arthrodesis. Current evidence shows possible increased healing rates and acceleration of healing times, especially in high-risk patients. Further randomized trials may be needed to focus on bone growth stimulation in the treatment of nonunions after foot and ankle arthrodesis and to determine which specific modality is most effective in treating foot and ankle nonunions.

REFERENCES

1. Griffin XL, Warner F, Costa M. The role of electromagnetic stimulation in the management of established non-union of long bone fractures: what is the evidence? Injury 2008;39(4):419–29.
2. Lente RW. Cases of un-united fracture treated by electricity. N Y State J Med 1850;5:317–9.
3. Hartshorne E. Pseudoarthroses. Am J Med Sci 1981;63:847–51.
4. Fukada E, Yasuda I. On the piezoelectric effect of bone. J Phys Soc Japan 1957; 12:1158–69.
5. Novicoff WM, Manaswi A, Hogan MV, et al. Critical analysis of the evidence for current technologies in bone-healing and repair. J Bone Joint Surg Am 2008; 90(Suppl 1):85–91.
6. Mollon B, da Silva V, Busse JW, et al. Electrical stimulation for long-bone fracture-healing: a meta-analysis of randomized controlled trials. J Bone Joint Surg Am 2008;90:2322–30.
7. Walker NA, Denegar CR, Preische J. Low-intensity pulsed ultrasound and pulsed electromagnetic field in the treatment of tibial fractures: a systematic review. J Athl Train 2007;42(4):530–5.
8. Kesani AK, Gandhi A, Lin SS. Electrical bone stimulation devices in foot and ankle surgery: types of devices, scientific basis, and clinical indications for their use. Foot Ankle Int 2006;27(2):148–56.
9. Schubert T, Kleditzsch J, Wolf E. Results of fluorescence microscopy studies of bone healing by direct stimulation with bipolar impulse currents and with the interference current procedure in the animal experiment. Z Orthop Ihre Grenzgeb 1986;124:6–12.
10. Reger SI, Hyodo A, Negami S, et al. Experimental wound healing with electrical stimulation. Artif Organs 1999;23:460–2.
11. Ohashi T. Electrical callus formation and its osteogenesis. Nippon Seikeigeka Gakkai Zasshi 1982;56(7):615–33.
12. Aaron RK, Ciombor DM, Keeping H, et al. Power frequency fields promote cell differentiation coincident with an increase in transforming growth factor-beta(1) expression. Bioelectromagnetics 1999;20:453–8.
13. Brighton CT, Wang W, Seldes R, et al. Signal transduction in electrically stimulated bone cells. J Bone Joint Surg Am 2001;83:1514–23.
14. Reher P, Harris M, Whiteman M, et al. Ultrasound stimulates nitric oxide and prostaglandin E2 production by human osteoblasts. Bone 2002;31:236–41.
15. Khan Y, Laurencin CT. Fracture repair with ultrasound: clinical and cell-based evaluation. J Bone Joint Surg Am 2008;90:138–44.
16. Hou C, Lin J, Huang S, et al. Ultrasound stimulates NF-kB activation and iNOS expression via the Ras/Raf/MEK/ERK signaling pathway in cultured preosteoblasts. J Cell Physiol 2009;220:196–203.
17. Wiss DA, Stetson WB. Tibial nonunion: treatment alternatives. J Am Acad Orthop Surg 1996;4(5):249–57.
18. Weber BG, Cech O. Pseudoarthrosis: pathology, biomechanics, therapy, results. Berne (Switzerland): Hans Huber; 1976.
19. Paterson D. Treatment of nonunion with a constant direct current: a totally implantable system. Orthop Clin North Am 1984;15:47–59.
20. Petersson CJ, Johnell O. Electrical stimulation of osteogenesis in delayed union of the rabbit fibula. Arch Orthop Trauma Surg 1983;101:247–50.

21. Kleczynski S. Electrical stimulation to promote the union of fractures. Int Orthop 1988;12:83–7.
22. Brighton CT, Black J, Friedenberg ZB, et al. A multicenter study of the treatment of non-union with constant direct current. J Bone Joint Surg Am 1981;63:2–13.
23. Ahl T, Andersson G, Herberts P, et al. Electrical treatment of non-united fractures. Acta Orthop Scand 1984;55:585–8.
24. Paterson DC, Lewis GN, Cass CA. Treatment of delayed union and nonunion with an implanted direct current stimulator. Clin Orthop 1980;148:117–28.
25. Brighton CT, Pollack SR. Treatment of recalcitrant non-union with a capacitively coupled electrical field. A preliminary report. J Bone Joint Surg Am 1985;67: 577–85.
26. Scott G, King JB. A prospective, double-blind trial of electrical capacitative coupling in the treatment of non-union of long bones. J Bone Joint Surg Am 1994;76:820–6.
27. Sarmiento A, Gersten LM, Sobol PA, et al. Tibial shaft fractures treated with functional braces. Experience with 780 fractures. J Bone Joint Surg Br 1989;71: 602–9.
28. Aaron RK, Ciombor DM, Simon BJ. Treatment of nonunions with electric and electromagnetic fields. Clin Orthop Relat Res 2004;419:21–9.
29. Bassett CA, Mitchell SN, Gaston SR. Pulsing electromagnetic field treatment in ununited fractures and failed arthrodeses. JAMA 1982;247:623–8.
30. Ibiwoye MO, Powell KA, Grabiner MD, et al. Bone mass is preserved in a critical-sized osteotomy by low energy pulsed electromagnetic fields as quantitated by in vivo micro-computed tomography. J Orthop Res 2004;22:1086–93.
31. Heckman JD, Ingram AJ, Loyd RD, et al. Nonunion treatment with pulsed electromagnetic fields. Clin Orthop Relat Res 1981;161:58–66.
32. Sharrard WJ. A double-blind trial of pulsed electromagnetic fields for delayed union of tibial fractures. J Bone Joint Surg Br 1990;72:347–55.
33. Bassett CA, Mitchell SN, Gaston SR. Treatment of ununited tibial diaphyseal fractures with pulsing electromagnetic fields. J Bone Joint Surg Am 1981;63: 511–23.
34. Fox IM, Smith SD. Bioelectric repair of metatarsal nonunions. J Foot Surg 1983; 22(2):108–15.
35. Holmes GB Jr. Treatment of delayed unions and nonunions of the proximal fifth metatarsal with pulsed electromagnetic fields. Foot Ankle Int 1994;15:552–6.
36. Fitzsimmons RJ, Ryaby JT, Mohan S, et al. Combined magnetic fields increase insulin-like growth factor-II in TE-85 human osteosarcoma bone cell cultures. Endocrinology 1995;136(7):3100–6.
37. Fitzsimmons RJ, Ryaby JT, Magee FP, et al. IGF-II receptor number is increased in TE-85 osteosarcoma cells by combined magnetic fields. J Bone Miner Res 1995;10(5):812–9.
38. Linovitz RJ, Pathria M, Bernhardt M, et al. Combined magnetic fields accelerate and increase spine fusion: a double-blind, randomized, placebo controlled study. Spine 2002;27(13):1383–9.
39. Hanft JR, Goggin JP, Landsman A, et al. The role of combined magnetic field bone growth stimulation as an adjunct in the treatment of neuroarthropathy/Charcot joint: an expanded pilot study. J Foot Ankle Surg 1998;37(6):510–5.
40. Papatheodorou LK, Malizos KN, Poultsides LA, et al. Effect of transosseous application of low-intensity ultrasound at the tendon graft-bone interface healing: gene expression and histological analysis in rabbits. Ultrasound Med Biol 2009;35(4): 576–84.

41. Duarte LR. The stimulation of bone growth by ultrasound. Arch Orthop Trauma Surg 1983;101:153–9.
42. Pilla AA, Mont M, Nasser PR, et al. Non-invasive low-intensity pulsed ultrasound accelerates bone healing in the rabbit. J Orthop Trauma 1990;4:246–53.
43. Takikawa S, Matsui N, Kokubu T, et al. Low-intensity pulsed ultrasound initiates bone healing in rat nonunion fracture model. J Ultrasound Med 2001;20:197–205.
44. Xavier CAM, Duarte LR. Estimulação ultrasônica do calo ósseo: aplicação clínica [Ultrasonic stimulation of bone callus: clinical application]. Rev Brasileira Orthop 1983;18:73–80 [in Portuguese].
45. Strauss E, Gonya G. Adjunct low intensity ultrasound in Charcot neuroarthropathy. Clin Orthop 1998;349:132–8.
46. Heckman JD, Ryaby JP, McCabe J, et al. Acceleration of tibial fracture-healing by non-invasive, low-intensity pulsed ultrasound. J Bone Joint Surg Am 1994;76: 26–34.
47. Cohen M, Roman A, Lovins JE. Totally implanted direct current stimulator as treatment for a nonunion in the foot. J Foot Ankle Surg 1993;32(4):375–81.
48. Donley BG, Ward DM. Implantable electrical stimulation in high-risk hindfoot fusions. Foot Ankle Int 2002;23(1):13–8.
49. Saxena A, DiDomenico LA, Widtfeldt A, et al. Implantable electrical bone stimulation for arthrodesis of the foot and ankle in high-risk patients: a multicenter study. J Foot Ankle Surg 2005;44(6):450–4.
50. Dhawan SK, Conti SF, Towers J, et al. The effect of pulsed electromagnetic fields on hindfoot arthrodesis: a prospective study. J Foot Ankle Surg 2004;43(2):93–6.
51. Midis N, Conti SF. Revision ankle arthrodesis. Foot Ankle Int 2002;23:243–7.
52. Saltzman C, Lightfoot A, Amendola A. PEMF as treatment for delayed healing of foot and ankle arthrodesis. Foot Ankle Int 2004;25:771–3.
53. Petrisor B, Lau JT. Electrical bone stimulation: an overview and its use in high risk and Charcot foot and ankle reconstructions. Foot Ankle Clin 2005;10(4):609–20.
54. Lau JT, Stamatis ED, Myerson MS, et al. Implantable direct-current bone stimulators in high-risk and revision foot and ankle surgery: a retrospective analysis with outcome assessment. Am J Orthop 2007;36(7):354–7.
55. Hockenbury RT, Gruttadauria M, McKinney I. Use of implantable bone growth stimulation in Charcot ankle arthrodesis. Foot Ankle Int 2007;28(9):971–6.
56. Jones CP, Coughlin MJ, Shurnas PS. Prospective CT scan evaluation of hindfoot nonunions treated with revision surgery and low-intensity ultrasound stimulation. Foot Ankle Int 2006;27(4):229–35.
57. Coughlin MJ, Smith BW, Traughber P. The evaluation of the healing rate of subtalar arthrodesis, part 2: the effect of low-intensity ultrasound stimulation. Foot Ankle Int 2008;29(10):970–7.

An Overview of Negative Pressure Wound Therapy for the Lower Extremity

Claire M. Capobianco, DPM, Thomas Zgonis, DPM, FACFAS*

KEYWORDS

- Negative pressure wound therapy • Diabetic ulcers
- Diabetic foot • Lower extremity • Diabetic neuropathy

Negative pressure wound therapy (NPWT) was originally introduced in the form of the now-ubiquitous Wound VAC by Kinetic Concepts, Inc. (San Antonio, TX) in 1995. The technology consists of computer-controlled application of subatmospheric pressure to a wound via a reticulated hydrophobic polyurethane or polyvinyl alcohol sponge under an occlusive dressing, with subsequent removal of wound exudate by an electromechanical pump. The technology has been widely embraced in surgical and surgical subspecialty arenas, and is used worldwide. The device is used in acute and chronic[1–5] wounds, on adults and children,[6] and in inpatient and outpatient[7,8] settings. A growing literature base has demonstrated largely positive results after use of NPWT, but, like any technology, it is not without controversy.

Most literature specific to the lower extremity focuses on the use of NPWT for diabetic ulcerations,[2,7,9–22] infected[23,24] and noninfected dehiscences,[23,25,26] skin grafting,[27–31] trauma,[32–43] and pressure ulcers.[44,45] In addition, NPWT has been used for wounds with compromised vascularity,[46] contaminated soft tissue injuries,[47] burns,[48–50] necrotizing fasciitis,[51–53] flaps and free tissue transfer,[54,55] calciphylaxis,[56] venomous[57] and nonvenomous[58] bite injuries, post-transplant wound infection,[59] eumycotic mycetoma,[60] malignant wounds,[61] pyoderma gangrenosum,[62,63] lymphocoeles,[64] lower extremity salvage,[65] venous stasis ulcers,[66] chronic osteomyelitis,[67,68] periprosthetic infections of hip and knee arthroplasties,[69] postmalignancy irradiation-induced ulcers,[70] combat-related soft tissue wounds,[47,71,72] infected wounds with exposed orthopedic implants,[73] chronic mycobacterial wound infection[74] over external fixation devices,[75] and with concurrent bone transport.[76]

Division of Podiatric Medicine and Surgery, Department of Orthopaedic Surgery, The University of Texas Health Science Center at San Antonio, San Antonio, Texas, USA
* Corresponding author
E-mail address: zgonis@uthscsa.edu (T. Zgonis).

Clin Podiatr Med Surg 26 (2009) 619–631
doi:10.1016/j.cpm.2009.08.002
0891-8422/09/$ – see front matter © 2009 Elsevier Inc. All rights reserved.

Currently, there are only a few brands of NPWT devices available in the United States, and their recommended pressure settings vary between 40 to 80 mm Hg and 125 mm Hg.[77,78] The initial cost and cost per day of these brands varies with insurance, but is comparable.

BACKGROUND AND MECHANISMS OF ACTION

The popularized mechanisms of action of NPWT are widely accepted and conceptually sound but also not without controversy. Subatmospheric pressure application causes physical contraction of complicated wounds and removes toxins, excess interstitial fluid, and slough from the wound bed, thereby optimizing the wound environment for angiogenesis and resultant granulation tissue formation. The effects of NPWT have been shown in one animal study to penetrate to a depth of only 1 mm in rabbit soft tissue.[79]

The mechanical effects of NPWT on wounds have been well studied in animal and computational models.[80,81] Foam sponge compressed by suction has been shown to induce microdeformations of the wound surface, which result in increased cell proliferation and the stimulation of angiogenesis.[82] Varying wound surface dressing types have been shown to affect these three-dimensional tissue microdeformations.[81] In the 1980s, a review article by Urschel and colleagues showed that mechanical stresses affect cellular proliferation in wounds.[3,83] Conversely, Nishimura and colleagues[84] reported a decrease in fibroblast proliferation and survival in a cellular model during high-frequency and intermittent tensile strain conditions.

Evaluation of biochemical markers in wound fluid has also shown interesting results. A rodent model demonstrated increased levels of vascular endothelial growth factor (VEGF), and fibroblast growth factor 2.[85] In human trauma patients, significantly increased levels of interleukin 8 (IL-8) and VEGF were noted in patients treated with NPWT compared with controls.[86] Reduced levels of hypoxia-induced factor 1α, an indirect marker of tissue oxygenation, were noted in patients with postirradiation ulcers treated by NPWT.[87] In a separate study, significantly reduced levels of matrix metalloproteases were found in wounds following NPWT treatment for 10 days.[88] Genetic data in rats have also shown increased expression of pathways involving inflammation and angiogenesis in subjects treated with NPWT versus controls.[89]

In addition, NPWT is believed to decrease the bacterial bioburden in wound beds via the application of continuous suction. An animal-model study in 1997 by Morykwas and colleagues[90] supported this hypothesis by demonstrating a significant decrease in tissue bacterial counts after 4 days of continuous application at 125 mm Hg. Furthermore, the closed wound environment and less frequent dressing changes (with less resultant potential exposure to new pathogens) also supports the theory of decreasing bioburden with NPWT.

CONTRAINDICATIONS FOR USE

A review of the current NPWT literature revealed the following contraindications: the devices are not intended for use over anastomoses, untreated osteomyelitis, malignancy (except for palliative care), unexplored fistulas, exposed organs, blood vessels, major structures, or necrotic tissue with eschar present.[77,78] In addition, malnourished patients are not appropriate candidates for NPWT secondary to presumed concern over insufficient baseline wound healing ability or the effect of decreased plasma albumin on wound fluid dynamics. Caution is recommended with NPWT use in the following patient subsets: those with marginal or difficult wound hemostasis, those who are anticoagulated, or those taking platelet aggregation inhibitors. The use of

NPWT over open cancelleous bone, as in a partial calcanectomy, is also debatable secondary to a presumed bleeding risk.

REPORTED COMPLICATIONS

Wound edge maceration and breakdown is likely the most common complication with NPWT, and is usually avoidable with careful sponge application, periwound skin protection, and barrier pastes. Premature discontinuation of therapy secondary to patient noncompliance, tube blockages, or adhesive tape reactions are also possible. In small-diameter wounds, the commonly used KCI TRAC pad has been shown to cause a localized pressure necrosis of surrounding fragile skin if the size of the wound is smaller than the area of the TRAC pad.[91] Easy application modifications alleviate this complication: the wound can be bordered by a hydrocolloid barrier; an extra piece of foam can be cut larger than the TRAC pad and stacked on top of the already sealed wound-foam-occlusive dressing construct; or the TRAC pad itself can be cut to a smaller size, so it is clear of any wound margins.

In large or complex wounds with sinus tracts and tunnels, the retained sponge is another potential complication.[92] For this reason, many health care professionals have taken to making a diagram of the number and location of sponges in any given wound type, and attaching this diagram to the tubing itself.

A case study detailing an unusual case of acquired hypoalbuminemia resulting in anasarca during NPWT was reported in 2005.[93] After ruling out other potential causes, the investigators concluded that the egress of the interstitial wound fluid via NPWT concomitantly removed clinically significant amounts of electrolytes and albumin in their patient. As a result, the investigators advise careful monitoring of patients with large surface area wounds, those who are elderly or debilitated, and those who have congestive heart failure.[93] In addition, although no formal case reports have been published to our knowledge, careful monitoring is also warranted to avoid inadvertent exsanguination for patients on anticoagulant therapy, platelet aggregate inhibitors, or those with marginal wound hemostasis.

ADVANTAGES

The widespread use of NPWT throughout multiple surgical disciplines and multiple wound types inherently compliments the technology's benefits. NPWT has been adopted by so many because the application of subatmospheric pressure in this fashion has been shown to maintain a moist wound healing environment, promote granulation tissue formation and wound contraction, and remove exudate and slough from the wound bed.[77,78] The interstitial fluid in chronic wounds is known to be rich in matrix metalloproteases and the removal of this fluid via NPWT is believed to help rebalance the biochemical environment of the wound, and allow for more efficient capillary microcirculation. In addition, compared with standard dressings, NPWT has been shown to specifically and significantly increase the cytokine IL-8 and VEGF concentrations in post-traumatic wounds.[86]

Studies also support the hypothesis that NPWT increases blood flow to the wound bed. Morykwas and colleagues[90,94] demonstrated, in 2 separate swine studies, that pressures of 125 mm Hg increased wound bed blood flow and, as a result, the investigators recommended this level of pressure for clinical application.

Conceptually, as previously described, NPWT is believed to decrease bacterial bioburden in the wound environment better than standard moist dressings. In addition, as previously described, the mechanical forces on wounds treated with NPWT are believed to benefit wound closure via physical wound contraction and proliferative cellular response to mechanical stresses. These stresses are believed to be different from those induced by surface debridement induced by removal of moist wound dressings.

Another advantage of NPWT is trauma-specific. This technology has been adopted as a temporizing dressing for open fractures and soft-tissue defects for the first 7 days, until definitive soft coverage can be obtained, and an early study suggests superiority of NPWT, compared with standard dressings, in these wounds. Fourteen of the 16 wounds included in this study were in the lower extremity.[86]

Another key advantage of NPWT is the ease of application and use, and the ability of home nursing to continue dressing changes after the patient is discharged from the hospital. Less frequent dressing changes result in less nursing time spent on dressing changes, which ultimately results in savings to the institution.

Multiple cost-effectiveness studies have been published that support the use of NPWT. Recently, Apelqvist and colleagues evaluated resource use and cost for 162 diabetic patients with postamputation pedal wounds and discovered significantly fewer reoperations and significantly fewer outpatient treatment visits in the NPWT group, compared with the moist dressing group. The average cost to 100% wound healing was approximately $12,000 more in the moist dressing group than the NPWT group, although this difference was not subject to statistical evaluation.[9] A retrospective study evaluating the incidence of diabetic foot amputations after treatment by NPWT versus traditional therapy showed significantly fewer amputations after use of NPWT. This finding was only significant in the Medicare cohort (n = 12,795), not in the private payer cohort (n = 3524),[15] and has been disputed.[22]

Another study evaluated the cost-effectiveness of NPWT in postsurgical patients with acute wounds in long-term acute-care hospitals. The investigators described significantly faster rates of wound closure, and lower cost-per-cubic-centimeter volume reduction in the NPWT group, compared with the advanced moist dressing group.[25]

Cost-effectiveness in trauma patients has also been evaluated. In a study including acute traumatic upper and lower extremity, abdominal, cardiovascular, flap or graft, sternotomy, and fasciotomy wounds, the investigators concluded that early intervention (before the third day of hospitalization) with NPWT was statistically beneficial for the patients. NPWT, started within this time frame, resulted in significantly fewer hospitalization days, treatment days, and intensive care unit days. This result, in turn, led to significantly lower total treatment costs.[39] Older studies also report superior[95] or equivocal[96] cost-effectiveness data for NPWT than for moist wound therapy.

DISADVANTAGES AND CRITICISMS

The most significant disadvantage of NPWT is the cost and availability of the therapy for uninsured patients and patients in less medically sophisticated countries. For this reason, some studies have provided details on the use of locally available materials for application of suction to wounds under occlusive dressings.[97,98]

In addition, evidence from the animal-model study of Morykwas and colleagues[90] that suggested that NWPT promotes healing by decreasing bacterial clearance from wounds was countered by Weed[99] in a study of 25 patients. Despite positive wound healing outcomes, the serial quantitative bacterial cultures obtained in the study failed to demonstrate consistent improvement in bacterial clearance from wounds as a result of NWPT therapy. Furthermore, a statistically significant increase in bacterial colonization was noted in wounds that were treated with NPWT.[99]

Debate also exists regarding the mechanism of action of NPWT. The role of tissue pressure during NPWT was initially examined by Kairinos and colleagues[100] in an in vitro meat model. They reported an increase in tissue pressure that was proportionate to the amount of suction applied. These data countered the widely accepted paradigm that pressure gradients were the driving forces that facilitated egress of edema and bacteria, and promoted perfusion during NPWT.[100] The roles of tissue pressure and perfusion during NPWT were recently re-examined by the same author group in a 2-part analysis. In the first article, an intracranial pressure sensor was used to measure interstitial tissue pressure with increasing application of NPWT pressure in circumferential, noncircumferential, and cavity conditions over 48 hours. An increase in tissue pressure was reported in all 3 groups despite a decrease in air pressure in the foam dressing.[101] Their follow-up study, which was based on intact skin only, reiterated increased tissue pressure during NPWT. In addition, decreased perfusion was noted with increased suction pressure during NPWT via radioisotope imaging and transcutaneous partial pressure of oxygen ($TcPo_2$) measurements. Multiple contradictory studies addressing tissue pressure and perfusion have been published in the literature, most of which used laser-based Doppler measurements.[90,102,103] The investigators criticized the use of laser Doppler secondary to the substantial effect of blood velocity on the measurements.[104] As a result of their data, the investigators advised against application of NPWT to tissues with suboptimal perfusion.

In addition, researchers have evaluated the effects of NPWT on patients' overall clinical condition, aside from the progress or regress of their wounds. Pain and basic functional activities in patients undergoing NPWT were evaluated by Apostoli and Caula in Italy in 2008. They suggested that pain and the consumption of analgesic medications increased, whereas patient autonomy decreased, during use of NPWT.[105] Dressing changes can be painful to the sensate patient, but can be ameliorated by premedication with analgesics or direct injection of fast-acting local anesthetic, such as 1% lidocaine, into the sponge minutes before its removal. Of note, the sponge must be disconnected from suction before injection of local anesthetic.

Although pain is often evaluated, Keskin and colleagues[106] hypothesized that NPWT could affect patients' anxiety levels, which could also have negative psychological effects. Compared with a group of patients with similar traumatic wounds who underwent classic non-NPWT treatment, the NPWT patients demonstrated a statistically significant increase in scores on 2 separate anxiety evaluation tools. This short-term study evaluated the patients after only 10 days of NPWT, but the results detailed previously undescribed effects of NPWT.

In addition, Mendonca and colleagues evaluated the effects of NPWT on quality of life, as measured by the Cardiff Wound Impact Schedule. Physical symptoms, social functioning, well-being, and overall quality of life were evaluated, but no definitive conclusions could be drawn from their data. Significant worsening in global quality-of-life scores were noted in the surgical intervention group and, as expected, physical functioning was significantly impaired in ambulatory patients. No significant change in quality-of-life scores was found for the group using a portable NPWT system compared with the patients whose wounds healed.[107]

The role of NPWT in the setting of orthopedic trauma was recently analyzed by Bhattacharryya and colleagues. In a retrospective evaluation of 38 patients with Gustilo-Anderson grade IIIB open tibial wounds, the investigators noted that the use of NPWT failed to allow delayed (more than 7 days) soft tissue coverage of the open wounds without a concomitant increase in the rate of infection. For this reason, they did advocate NPWT as a temporary dressing for open tibial fractures, but also recommended early and definitive soft-tissue closure within 7 days of injury to reduce the risk of deep infection.[33]

Some investigators recognize the reported results of NPWT, but remain skeptical of comparative superiority to classic wound-care methods. They worry that the ease of use, and relative infrequency, of subsequent dressing changes may be inadequate reasons for the surgeon to wholeheartedly embrace the technology, and caution that significant unnoticed blood loss could result.[108]

EVALUATION OF THE PUBLISHED TRIALS

Multiple critical literature reviews and analyses of the evidence behind NPWT have been published in the past 5 years.[2,4,5,20,38,50,109] A comprehensive evaluation of these metareviews is beyond the scope of this article, but salient points are emphasized from the most thorough of these analyses. A comprehensive evaluation of 7 randomized controlled trials (RCTs) and 10 non-RCTs performed by Gregor and colleagues in 2008 demonstrated significant differences in time to, or incidence of, wound closure in almost 50% of the studies examined. In addition, a meta-analysis for change in wound size supported NPWT use. However, the investigators were unimpressed by the overall quality of methodology in the 17 studies included in the analysis. They reported evidence of 8 unpublished or prematurely terminated NPWT trials, which they felt was cause for concern.[110]

A Cochrane analysis in 2008, authored by Ubbink and colleagues,[3] on NPWT and chronic wounds reported somewhat different conclusions. Seven trials involving 205 patients were included in their analysis and the investigators concluded, based on the studies, that NPWT did not demonstrate a significant advantage on healing rates versus standard mixed wound care treatments (saline, papain-urea, cadhexamer iodine, hydrocolloids, foams, and hydrogels). These investigators ultimately conceded that NPWT does demonstrate a beneficial effect on the healing of chronic wounds but also criticized the poor methodology of the studies and recommended better powered and better designed studies.

The other Cochrane analysis for NPWT is specific for use on partial thickness burns. However, only 1 study met the inclusion criteria of the investigators, and it was underpowered and lacking design finesse, so they conceded that any meaningful conclusions could not be drawn because of the lack of well-designed studies.[50]

Hinchliffe and colleagues[2] undertook a systematic review of the use of NPWT and multiple other therapies including larvae, sharp debridement, antiseptic use, hyperbaric oxygen, hydrogels, skin grafts, ultrasound, and electric stimulation for the diabetic foot. Sixty articles met their inclusion criteria. They concluded that NPWT "may promote healing of post-operative wounds." Kanakaris and colleagues[38] reviewed 16 studies regarding traumatic application of NPWT, and concluded that effectiveness was comparable to standard wound coverage and dressings, and that the evidence justified the application of NPWT to lower-extremity injuries with soft tissue trauma.

RECENT ADVANCES

The advent of competition in the NPWT market will likely coincide with continued innovation on the part of the manufacturers. Recently, silver-impregnated foams were introduced with the intention of more efficient moderation of the bacterial population in the wound. Attention has also been paid to design updates to the foam and occlusive dressing materials to minimize the time required to customize those products to individual wounds. In addition, specialized prefabricated bridging devices have been introduced that are also intended to minimize time spent on more complex lower extremity wounds.

In contrast, other manufacturers advertise a lower pressure setting on their devices (40–80 mm Hg) for the benefit of painless treatment. Their devices are able to apply 125 mm Hg, but, currently, their clinical guidelines recommend the lower settings. In addition, the devices are approved to work with reticulated foam or gauze base dressings. The use of gauze dressings has been evaluated in small studies and, to date, comparable outcomes have been reported.[111] Early studies evaluating different topical interfaces suggest that more research is needed in this particular subfield.[112]

In addition, coordinating irrigation and instillation therapy have become more popular with the use of NPWT. Results using irrigation have been reported for infected wounds and ulcers[113–116] and osteomyelitis,[68] although doubt exists on the effectiveness of this technique to irrigate the entire wound surface.[117]

SUMMARY

Published evidence continues to support the use of NPWT in multiple applications. In the lower extremity, techniques of managing traumatic, diabetic, postsurgical, and peripheral vascular disease–associated wounds with NPWT continue to advance. More quality, randomized, controlled trials are needed for better understanding of the appropriate scope and effects of this technology, and for further elucidation of its mechanisms of action.

REFERENCES

1. Evans D, Land L. Topical negative pressure for treating chronic wounds: a systematic review. Br J Plast Surg 2001;54(3):238–42.
2. Hinchliffe RJ, Valk GD, Apelqvist J, et al. A systematic review of the effectiveness of interventions to enhance the healing of chronic ulcers of the foot in diabetes. Diabetes Metab Res Rev 2008;24(Suppl1):S119–44.
3. Ubbink DT, Westerbos SJ, Evans D, et al. Topical negative pressure for treating chronic wounds. Cochrane Database Syst Rev 2008;(3):CD001898.
4. Ubbink DT, Westerbos SJ, Nelson EA, et al. A systematic review of topical negative pressure therapy for acute and chronic wounds. Br J Surg 2008;95(6): 685–92.
5. Vig S. A systematic review of topical negative pressure therapy for acute and chronic wounds. Br J Surg 2008;95:685–92 Br J Surg 2008;95(9):1185–6; author reply 1186.
6. Caniano DA, Ruth B, Teich S. Wound management with vacuum-assisted closure: experience in 51 pediatric patients. J Pediatr Surg 2005;40(1):128–32.
7. Fife CE, Walker D, Thomson B, et al. The safety of negative pressure wound therapy using vacuum-assisted closure in diabetic foot ulcers treated in the outpatient setting. Int Wound J 2008;5(Suppl 2):17–22.
8. Sibbald RG, Woo KY. V.A.C. therapy in home care. Int Wound J 2008;5(Suppl 2): iii–iv.
9. Apelqvist J, Armstrong DG, Lavery LA, et al. Resource utilization and economic costs of care based on a randomized trial of vacuum-assisted closure therapy in the treatment of diabetic foot wounds. Am J Surg 2008;195(6):782–8.
10. Armstrong DG, Lavery LA, Diabetic Foot Study C. Negative pressure wound therapy after partial diabetic foot amputation: a multicentre, randomised controlled trial. Lancet 2005;366(9498):1704–10.

11. Blume PA, Walters J, Payne W, et al. Comparison of negative pressure wound therapy using vacuum-assisted closure with advanced moist wound therapy in the treatment of diabetic foot ulcers: a multicenter randomized controlled trial. Diabetes Care 2008;31(4):631–6.

12. Dougherty EJ. An evidence-based model comparing the cost-effectiveness of platelet-rich plasma gel to alternative therapies for patients with nonhealing diabetic foot ulcers. Adv Skin Wound Care 2008;21(12):568–75.

13. Eneroth M, van Houtum WH. The value of debridement and vacuum-assisted closure (V.A.C.) therapy in diabetic foot ulcers. Diabetes Metab Res Rev 2008;24(Suppl 1):S76–80.

14. Flack S, Apelqvist J, Keith M, et al. An economic evaluation of VAC therapy compared with wound dressings in the treatment of diabetic foot ulcers. J Wound Care 2008;17(2):71–8.

15. Frykberg RG, Williams DV. Negative-pressure wound therapy and diabetic foot amputations: a retrospective study of payer claims data. J Am Podiatr Med Assoc 2007;97(5):351–9.

16. Hemkens LG, Waltering A. Comparison of negative pressure wound therapy using vacuum-assisted closure with advanced moist wound therapy in the treatment of diabetic foot ulcers: a multicenter randomized controlled trial: response to Blume et al. Diabetes Care 2008;31(10):e76 [author reply e77].

17. Lavery LA, Barnes SA, Keith MS, et al. Prediction of healing for postoperative diabetic foot wounds based on early wound area progression. Diabetes Care 2008;31(1):26–9.

18. Lavery LA, Boulton AJ, Niezgoda JA, et al. A comparison of diabetic foot ulcer outcomes using negative pressure wound therapy versus historical standard of care. Int Wound J 2007;4(2):103–13.

19. Maegele M, Gregor S, Peinemann F, et al. Negative pressure therapy in diabetic foot wounds. Lancet 2006;367(9512):725–6 [author reply 726–7].

20. Suess JJ, Kim PJ, Steinberg JS. Negative pressure wound therapy: evidence-based treatment for complex diabetic foot wounds. Curr Diab Rep 2006;6(6):446–50.

21. Tan D, Rajanayagam J, Schwarz F. Treatment of long-standing, poor-healing diabetic foot ulcers with topical negative pressure in the Torres Strait. Aust J Rural Health 2007;15(4):275–6.

22. Udell E. Negative-pressure wound therapy and diabetic foot amputations: a retrospective study of Payer Claims Data. J Am Podiatr Med Assoc 2008; 98(2):164–5 author reply 165.

23. Howell-Taylor M, Hall MG Jr, Brownlee Iii WJ, et al. Negative pressure wound therapy combined with acoustic pressure wound therapy for infected post surgery wounds: a case series. Ostomy Wound Manage 2008;54(9):49–52.

24. Wongworawat MD, Schnall SB, Holtom PD, et al. Negative pressure dressings as an alternative technique for the treatment of infected wounds. Clin Orthop Relat Res 2003;(414):45–8.

25. de Leon JM, Barnes S, Nagel M, et al. Cost-effectiveness of negative pressure wound therapy for postsurgical patients in long-term acute care. Adv Skin Wound Care 2009;22(3):122–7.

26. Ferdinando E, Guerin L, Jervis AO, et al. Negative-pressure wound therapy and external fixation for infection and hematoma after hallux abducto valgus surgery. J Am Podiatr Med Assoc 2007;97(5):410–4.

27. Blackburn JH 2nd, Boemi L, Hall WW, et al. Negative-pressure dressings as a bolster for skin grafts. Ann Plast Surg 1998;40(5):453–7.

28. Kim EK, Hong JP. Efficacy of negative pressure therapy to enhance take of 1-stage allodermis and a split-thickness graft. Ann Plast Surg 2007;58(5): 536–40.

29. Korber A, Franckson T, Grabbe S, et al. Vacuum assisted closure device improves the take of mesh grafts in chronic leg ulcer patients. Dermatology 2008;216(3):250–6.

30. Moisidis E, Heath T, Boorer C, et al. A prospective, blinded, randomized, controlled clinical trial of topical negative pressure use in skin grafting. Plast Reconstr Surg 2004;114(4):917–22.

31. Poulakidas S, Kowal-Vern A. Facilitating residual wound closure after partial graft loss with vacuum assisted closure therapy. J Burn Care Res 2008;29(4):663–5.

32. Bollero D, Carnino R, Risso D, et al. Acute complex traumas of the lower limbs: a modern reconstructive approach with negative pressure therapy. Wound Repair Regen 2007;15(4):589–94.

33. Bhattacharyya T, Mehta P, Smith M, et al. Routine use of wound vacuum-assisted closure does not allow coverage delay for open tibia fractures. Plast Reconstr Surg 2008;121(4):1263–6.

34. Brem MH, Blanke M, Olk A, et al. The vacuum-assisted closure (V.A.C.) and instillation dressing: limb salvage after 3 degrees open fracture with massive bone and soft tissue defect and superinfection. Unfallchirurg 2008;111(2):122–5 [in German].

35. Dedmond BT, Kortesis B, Punger K, et al. The use of negative-pressure wound therapy (NPWT) in the temporary treatment of soft-tissue injuries associated with high-energy open tibial shaft fractures. J Orthop Trauma 2007;21(1):11–7.

36. Goon PK, Dalal M. Limb-threatening extravasation injury: topical negative pressure and limb salvage. Plast Reconstr Surg 2006;117(3):1064–5.

37. Herscovici D Jr, Sanders RW, Scaduto JM, et al. Vacuum-assisted wound closure (VAC therapy) for the management of patients with high-energy soft tissue injuries. J Orthop Trauma 2003;17(10):683–8.

38. Kanakaris NK, Thanasas C, Keramaris N, et al. The efficacy of negative pressure wound therapy in the management of lower extremity trauma: review of clinical evidence. Injury 2007;38(Suppl 5):S9–18.

39. Kaplan M, Daly D, Stemkowski S. Early intervention of negative pressure wound therapy using vacuum-assisted closure in trauma patients: impact on hospital length of stay and cost. Adv Skin Wound Care 2009;22(3):128–32.

40. Rinker B, Amspacher JC, Wilson PC, et al. Subatmospheric pressure dressing as a bridge to free tissue transfer in the treatment of open tibia fractures. Plast Reconstr Surg 2008;121(5):1664–73.

41. Schlatterer D, Hirshorn K. Negative pressure wound therapy with reticulated open cell foam-adjunctive treatment in the management of traumatic wounds of the leg: a review of the literature. J Orthop Trauma 2008;22(Suppl 10): S152–160.

42. Stannard JP, Robinson JT, Anderson ER, et al. Negative pressure wound therapy to treat hematomas and surgical incisions following high-energy trauma. J Trauma 2006;60(6):1301–6.

43. Tarkin IS. The versatility of negative pressure wound therapy with reticulated open cell foam for soft tissue management after severe musculoskeletal trauma. J Orthop Trauma 2008;22(Suppl 10):S146–51.

44. Mandal A. Role of topical negative pressure in pressure ulcer management. J Wound Care 2007;16(1):33–5.

45. Niezgoda JA. Incorporating negative pressure therapy into the management strategy for pressure ulcers. Ostomy Wound Manage 2004;50(11A Suppl): 5S–8S.

46. Nordmyr J, Svensson S, Bjorck M, et al. Vacuum assisted wound closure in patients with lower extremity arterial disease. The experience from two tertiary referral-centres. Int Angiol 2009;28(1):26–31.

47. Leininger BE, Rasmussen TE, Smith DL, et al. Experience with wound VAC and delayed primary closure of contaminated soft tissue injuries in Iraq. J Trauma 2006;61(5):1207–11.

48. Schintler M, Marschitz I, Trop M. The use of topical negative pressure in a paediatric patient with extensive burns. Burns 2005;31(8):1050–3.

49. Terrazas SG. Adjuvant dressing for negative pressure wound therapy in burns. Ostomy Wound Manage 2006;52(1):16–8.

50. Wasiak J, Cleland H. Topical negative pressure (TNP) for partial thickness burns. Cochrane Database Syst Rev 2007;(3):CD006215.

51. Baharestani MM. Negative pressure wound therapy in the adjunctive management of necrotizing fasciitis: examining clinical outcomes. Ostomy Wound Manage 2008;54(4):44–50.

52. Martin DA, Nanci GN, Marlowe SI, et al. Necrotizing fasciitis with no mortality or limb loss. Am Surg 2008;74(9):809–12.

53. Steinstraesser L, Sand M, Steinau HU. Giant VAC in a patient with extensive necrotizing fasciitis. Int J Low Extrem Wounds 2009;8(1):28–30.

54. Bannasch H, Iblher N, Penna V, et al. A critical evaluation of the concomitant use of the implantable Doppler probe and the vacuum assisted closure system in free tissue transfer. Microsurgery 2008;28(6):412–6.

55. Uygur F, Duman H, Ulkur E, et al. The role of the vacuum-assisted closure therapy in the salvage of venous congestion of the free flap: case report. Int Wound J 2008;5(1):50–3.

56. Strippoli D, Simonetti V, Russo G, et al. Calciphylaxis: a case report. Dermatol Ther 2008;21(Suppl 3):S26–28.

57. Miller MS, Ortegon M, McDaniel C. Negative pressure wound therapy: treating a venomous insect bite. Int Wound J 2007;4(1):88–92.

58. Donate G, Emerick Salas R, Naidu D, et al. Nonvenomous bite injuries of the foot: case reports and review of the literature. Int J Low Extrem Wounds 2008; 7(1):41–4.

59. Shrestha BM, Nathan VC, Delbridge MC, et al. Vacuum-assisted closure (VAC) therapy in the management of wound infection following renal transplantation. Kathmandu Univ Med J (KUMJ) 2007;5(1):4–7.

60. Estrada-Chavez GE, Vega-Memije ME, Arenas R, et al. Eumycotic mycetoma caused by Madurella mycetomatis successfully treated with antifungals, surgery, and topical negative pressure therapy. Int J Dermatol 2009;48(4):401–3.

61. Ford-Dunn S. Use of vacuum assisted closure therapy in the palliation of a malignant wound. Palliat Med 2006;20(4):477–8.

62. Geller SM, Longton JA. Ulceration of pyoderma gangrenosum treated with negative pressure wound therapy. J Am Podiatr Med Assoc 2005;95(2):171–4.

63. Ghersi MM, Ricotti C, Nousari CH, et al. Negative pressure dressing in the management of pyoderma gangrenosum ulcer. Arch Dermatol 2007;143(10): 1249–51.

64. Hamed O, Muck PE, Smith JM, et al. Use of vacuum-assisted closure (VAC) therapy in treating lymphatic complications after vascular procedures: new approach for lymphoceles. J Vasc Surg 2008;48(6):1520–3, 1523, e1521–4.

65. Horch RE, Dragu A, Lang W, et al. Coverage of exposed bones and joints in critically ill patients: lower extremity salvage with topical negative pressure therapy. J Cutan Med Surg 2008;12(5):223–9.
66. Loree S, Dompmartin A, Penven K, et al. Is vacuum assisted closure a valid technique for debriding chronic leg ulcers? J Wound Care 2004;13(6):249–52.
67. Lam WL, Garrido A, Stanley PR. Use of topical negative pressure in the treatment of chronic osteomyelitis. A case report. J Bone Joint Surg Am 2005; 87(3):622–4.
68. Timmers MS, Graafland N, Bernards AT, et al. Negative pressure wound treatment with polyvinyl alcohol foam and polyhexanide antiseptic solution instillation in posttraumatic osteomyelitis. Wound Repair Regen 2009;17(2):278–86.
69. Lehner B, Bernd L. V.A.C.-instill therapy in periprosthetic infection of hip and knee arthroplasty. Zentralbl Chir 2006;131(Suppl 1):S160–4 [in German].
70. Loos B, Kopp J, Hohenberger W, et al. Post-malignancy irradiation ulcers with exposed alloplastic materials can be salvaged with topical negative pressure therapy (TNP). Eur J Surg Oncol 2007;33(7):920–5.
71. Murray CK, Hsu JR, Solomkin JS, et al. Prevention and management of infections associated with combat-related extremity injuries. J Trauma 2008; 64(Suppl 3):S239–51.
72. Pirela-Cruz MA, Machen MS, Esquivel D. Management of large soft-tissue wounds with negative pressure therapy-lessons learned from the war zone. J Hand Ther 2008;21(2):196–202, quiz 203.
73. Pelham FR, Kubiak EN, Sathappan SS, et al. Topical negative pressure in the treatment of infected wounds with exposed orthopaedic implants. J Wound Care 2006;15(3):111–6.
74. Vigler M, Mulett H, Hausman MR. Chronic *Mycobacterium* infection of first dorsal web space after accidental Bacilli Calmette-Guerin injection in a health worker: case report. J Hand Surg [Am] 2008;33(9):1621–4.
75. Lemmon JA, Ahmad J, Ghavami A, et al. Vacuum-assisted closure over an external fixation device. Plast Reconstr Surg 2008;121(4):234e–5e.
76. Somanchi BV, Khan S. Vacuum-assisted wound closure (VAC) with simultaneous bone transport in the leg: a technical note. Acta Orthop Belg 2008;74(4):538–41.
77. Zgonis T, Stapleton JJ, Girard-Powell VA, et al. Surgical management of diabetic foot infections and amputations. AORN 2008;87(5):935–46.
78. Zgonis T, Stapleton JJ, Rodriguez RH, et al. Plastic surgery reconstruction of the diabetic foot. AORN 2008;87(5):951–66.
79. Murphey GC, Macias BR, Hargens AR. Depth of penetration of negative pressure wound therapy into underlying tissues. Wound Repair Regen 2009;17(1):113–7.
80. Malmsjo M, Ingemansson R, Martin R, et al. Negative-pressure wound therapy using gauze or open-cell polyurethane foam: similar early effects on pressure transduction and tissue contraction in an experimental porcine wound model. Wound Repair Regen 2009;17(2):200–5.
81. Wilkes R, Zhao Y, Kieswetter K, et al. Effects of dressing type on 3D tissue microdeformations during negative pressure wound therapy: a computational study. J Biomech Eng 2009;131(3):031012.
82. Scherer SS, Pietramaggiori G, Mathews JC, et al. The mechanism of action of the vacuum-assisted closure device. Plast Reconstr Surg 2008;122(3): 786–97.
83. Urschel JD, Scott PG, Williams HTG. The effect of mechanical stress on soft and hard tissue repair; a review. British Journal of Plastic Surgery 1988;42(2): 182–6.

84. Nishimura K, Blume P, Ohgi S, et al. Effect of different frequencies of tensile strain on human dermal fibroblast proliferation and survival. Wound Repair Regen 2007;15(5):646–56.

85. Jacobs S, Simhaee DA, Marsano A, et al. Efficacy and mechanisms of vacuum-assisted closure (VAC) therapy in promoting wound healing: a rodent model. J Plast Reconstr Aesthet Surg 2008 [epub ahead of print].

86. Labler L, Rancan M, Mica L, et al. Vacuum-assisted closure therapy increases local interleukin-8 and vascular endothelial growth factor levels in traumatic wounds. J Trauma 2009;66(3):749–57.

87. Grimm A, Dimmler A, Stange S, et al. Expression of HIF-1 alpha in irradiated tissue is altered by topical negative-pressure therapy. Strahlenther Onkol 2007;183(3):144–9.

88. Moues CM, van Toorenenbergen AW, Heule F, et al. The role of topical negative pressure in wound repair: expression of biochemical markers in wound fluid during wound healing. Wound Repair Regen 2008;16(4):488–94.

89. Derrick KL, Norbury K, Kieswetter K, et al. Comparative analysis of global gene expression profiles between diabetic rat wounds treated with vacuum-assisted closure therapy, moist wound healing or gauze under suction. Int Wound J 2008;5(5):615–24.

90. Morykwas MJ, Argenta LC, Shelton-Brown EI, et al. Vacuum-assisted closure: a new method for wound control and treatment: animal studies and basic foundation. Ann Plast Surg 1997;38(6):553–62.

91. Jones SM, Banwell PE, Shakespeare PG, et al. Complications of topical negative pressure therapy in small-diameter wounds. Plast Reconstr Surg 2004;114(3): 815–7.

92. Leijnen M, Steenvoorde P. A retained sponge is a complication of vacuum-assisted closure therapy. Int J Low Extrem Wounds 2008;7(1):51.

93. Friedman T, Westreich M, Shalom A. Vacuum-assisted closure treatment complicated by anasarca. Ann Plast Surg 2005;55(4):420–1.

94. Morykwas MJ, Faler BJ, Pearce DJ, et al. Effects of varying levels of subatmospheric pressure on the rate of granulation tissue formation in experimental wounds in swine. Ann Plast Surg 2001;47(5):547–51.

95. Neubauer G, Ujlaky R. The cost-effectiveness of topical negative pressure versus other wound-healing therapies. J Wound Care 2003;12(10):392–3.

96. Moues CM, van den Bemd GJ, Meerding WJ, et al. An economic evaluation of the use of TNP on full-thickness wounds. J Wound Care 2005;14(5):224–7.

97. Bui TD, Huerta S, Gordon IL. Negative pressure wound therapy with off-the-shelf components. Am J Surg 2006;192(2):235–7.

98. Shalom A, Eran H, Westreich M, et al. Our experience with a "homemade" vacuum-assisted closure system. Isr Med Assoc J 2008;10(8–9):613–6.

99. Weed T, Ratliff C, Drake DB. Quantifying bacterial bioburden during negative pressure wound therapy: does the wound VAC enhance bacterial clearance? Ann Plast Surg 2004;52(3):276–9 [discussion: 279–80].

100. Kairinos N, Solomons M, Hudson DA. The paradox of negative pressure wound therapy – in vitro studies. J Plast Reconstr Aesthet Surg 2008 [epub ahead of print].

101. Kairinos N, Solomons M, Hudson DA. Negative-pressure wound therapy I: the paradox of negative-pressure wound therapy. Plast Reconstr Surg 2009; 123(2):589–98 [discussion: 599–600].

102. Argenta LC, Morykwas MJ. Vacuum-assisted closure: a new method for wound control and treatment: clinical experience. Ann Plast Surg 1997;38(6):563–76 [discussion: 577].
103. Wackenfors A, Sjogren J, Gustafsson R, et al. Effects of vacuum-assisted closure therapy on inguinal wound edge microvascular blood flow. Wound Repair Regen 2004;12(6):600–6.
104. Kairinos N, Voogd AM, Botha PH, et al. Negative-pressure wound therapy II: negative-pressure wound therapy and increased perfusion. Just an illusion? Plast Reconstr Surg 2009;123(2):601–12.
105. Apostoli A, Caula C. Pain and basic functional activities in a group of patients with cutaneous wounds under V.A.C therapy in hospital setting. Prof Inferm 2008;61(3):158–64 [in Italian].
106. Keskin M, Karabekmez FE, Yilmaz E, et al. Vacuum-assisted closure of wounds and anxiety. Scand J Plast Reconstr Surg Hand Surg 2008;42(4):202–5.
107. Mendonca DA, Drew PJ, Harding KG, et al. A pilot study on the effect of topical negative pressure on quality of life. J Wound Care 2007;16(2):49–53.
108. Greenhalgh DG. Negative pressure therapy, a panacea or not? Wound Repair Regen 2007;15(4):433.
109. Vikatmaa P, Juutilainen V, Kuukasjarvi P, et al. Negative pressure wound therapy: a systematic review on effectiveness and safety. Eur J Vasc Endovasc Surg 2008;36(4):438–48.
110. Gregor S, Maegele M, Sauerland S, et al. Negative pressure wound therapy: a vacuum of evidence? Arch Surg 2008;143(2):189–96.
111. Campbell PE, Smith GS, Smith JM. Retrospective clinical evaluation of gauze-based negative pressure wound therapy. Int Wound J 2008;5(2):280–6.
112. Jones SM, Banwell PE, Shakespeare PG. Interface dressings influence the delivery of topical negative-pressure therapy. Plast Reconstr Surg 2005;116(4):1023–8.
113. Chien SH, Tan WH, Hsu H. New continuous negative-pressure and irrigation treatment for infected wounds and intractable ulcers. Plast Reconstr Surg 2008;122(1):318 [author reply 319].
114. Gabriel A, Shores J, Heinrich C, et al. Negative pressure wound therapy with instillation: a pilot study describing a new method for treating infected wounds. Int Wound J 2008;5(3):399–413.
115. Jerome D. Advances in negative pressure wound therapy: the VAC instill. J Wound Ostomy Continence Nurs 2007;34(2):191–4.
116. Kiyokawa K, Takahashi N, Rikimaru H, et al. New continuous negative-pressure and irrigation treatment for infected wounds and intractable ulcers. Plast Reconstr Surg 2007;120(5):1257–65.
117. Lee SS, Chang KP, Lai CS, et al. Does continuous negative-pressure and irrigation treatment really rinse the whole closed wound? Plast Reconstr Surg 2008;122(1):319–20 [author reply 320–11].

Current Concepts and Techniques
in Foot and Ankle Surgery

Biologic Resurfacing of the Ankle and First Metatarsophalangeal Joint: Case Studies with a 2-Year Follow-Up

Stephen A. Brigido, DPM[a],*, Michael Troiano, DPM[b],
Harold Schoenhaus, DPM[b]

KEYWORDS

- Biologic resurfacing • Acellular regenerative tissue scaffold
- Ankle arthritis • First metatarsophalangeal joint arthritis
- Arthrodiastasis

CUTIS ARTHROPLASTY: A HISTORICAL PERSPECTIVE

Since the nineteenth century, arthroplasty has been a favored solution for patients with problem joints; however, the nature of the interposing material has often perplexed surgeons. In the past, rather than look within the body itself for a viable membrane, researchers sought and produced artificial materials—chromicized pig bladder by Baer[1] in 1918, cellophane by McKeever[2] in 1943, and nylon by Burman[3] in 1943. From 1920 to 1940, fascia lata became the most commonly used material. Fascia lata was preferred because of its acceptability to its host, but it was not without drawbacks: limited supply, lack of pliability, and susceptibility to tearing.[4] The cutis, or dermal graft, seemed to offer all of the benefits of fascia lata with none of the disadvantages; thus in the 1950s cutis began its reign as the interposing membrane of choice.

In 1956, Kettunen[5] studied the autogenous whole-thickness skin graft used as interposing material in hip-joint arthroplasties performed on 6 adult cats. The hip joint was opened with a lateral incision, and the interarticular cartilage was removed from the acetabulum. The skin graft was then placed into the joint—with the epidermal side

Conflicts: Stephen A. Brigido, DPM, and Harold Schoenhaus, DPM are consultants for Wright Medical Technology.

[a] Foot and Ankle Center at Coordinated Health, 2775 Schoenersville Road, Bethlehem, PA 18017, USA
[b] Penn-Presbyterian Medical Center, 1740 South Street, Suite 500, Philadelphia, PA 19146, USA
* Corresponding author.
E-mail address: drsbrigido@mac.com (S.A. Brigido).

Clin Podiatr Med Surg 26 (2009) 633–645
doi:10.1016/j.cpm.2009.07.005
0891-8422/09/$ – see front matter
© 2009 Elsevier Inc. All rights reserved.
podiatric.theclinics.com

against the surface of the acetabulum—and was attached by sutures. The leg was immobilized for 2 weeks, after which the cat was encouraged to move freely. On examination, the acetabulum revealed that the transplanted skin graft retained its vitality and developed new tendonlike connective tissue, acting as an organic layer between the joint surfaces.

A 1958 study on the use of cutis as an interposing membrane in knee arthroplasty on 4 patients had similar successful results. Realizing that the most satisfactory material is the deepest layer of the derma that contains a minimum amount of fat, Brown and colleagues[4] discovered that the easiest way to obtain this cutis was to use a dermatome. The graft was inserted into the joint, with the fatty tissue forming the new joint surface and the superficial layer adjacent to the bone. Using the "pull-out wire" technique, the graft was sutured at corners so that it was draped over bone surfaces. Wires were then tied under moderate tension over buttons on the skin surface. After all wires were inserted, excess graft was removed. A 3-week immobilization period was required to allow the graft to "take," after which physical therapy was progressively administered. All 4 arthroplasties were rated successful; the range of active motion varied from 60° to 80°, and extension of 180° was achieved in all cases.

Kelley and Gross[6] used a comparable technique with a hip-joint arthroplasty in 1958. A split-thickness graft was removed from the lower abdomen with a dermatome and left attached on one of its lateral borders. A dermal graft with a small amount of fat was then removed, and the split-thickness graft was sutured back to cover the abdomen. A Smith-Peterson incision was made, exposing the left hip anteriorly and superiorly, and the entire capsule was removed. The remnants of the capsule were excised, and the head of the femur was dislocated and trimmed to cancellous bleeding bone. The dermal graft was fitted over this bone and held by a circumferential purse-string suture. The head of the femur was then reduced to its original position. Although the patient was allowed to move his knee, ankle, and toes 24 hours after surgery, the hip was immobilized for approximately 1 month. A small infected area along the incision developed after 3 weeks; it was superficial and did not penetrate the fascia. The surgery was deemed successful, with a leg flexion of 90°, normal external rotation of 70°, normal internal rotation of 50°, and no pain in the hip joint.

From 1969 to 1971, Bailey[7] performed dermal arthroplasties on 30 hands severely crippled by rheumatoid arthritis. Dermis was cut from the submammary region where it is thickest, and an incision was made 3 mm radial to and parallel with the extensor tendon over the metacarpophalangeal joint. Dermis was cut into a 1- by 2-cm strip, and inserted into the artificial joint cavity as a double layer with the hinge ventral and the subepithelial layer of the dermis toward the bone ends. The graft was held into position by 3 fine nylon stitches through the periosteal cuff on the metacarpal neck and the base of the phalanx. The hood was closed with radial overlap, and the extensor indicis proprius was rerouted through the thumb web. All patients reported an absence of pain, and all but one felt they had better hand function. All patients with the exception of one made a large gain in joint range. One poor result with active flexion from 45° to 70° at all metacarpophalangeal joints followed a breakdown of a transverse wound, which occurred after 3 weeks. Two cases had a mild recurrence of proximal phalangeal subluxation at 1 and 2.5 years, respectively.

Froimson and colleagues[8] performed dermal arthroplasty of the elbow joint on 5 patients in 1976. A dermatome was used to remove a split-thickness skin graph, and the cutis graft was applied to the distal end of the humerus with the superficial side against the bone. The graft was sutured to the bone through 2 drill holes. The seams on either side of the graft were closed, trimming excess cutis to achieve a snug fit. The elbow was then reduced, and a compression dressing was applied.

A posterior plaster splint was used to immobilize the elbow in 90° flexion for 2 weeks; after which gentle exercises commenced (between the periods of exercise, the splint was reapplied). In all patients, a satisfactory excursion of flexion and extension was achieved, and pronation and supination were satisfactory.

Uuspää[9] achieved similar results when he performed 51 elbow arthroplasties between 1978 and 1984. Flexion contracture was diminished, and range of flexion and range of rotation were improved. Sixteen patients reported no pain, whereas others reported pain at times. Thirteen patients had ulnar nerve symptoms before arthroplasty, and only 2 of these had symptoms after surgery. In all, 8 patients had ulnar nerve symptoms after arthroplasty. In 5 of these, elbow joints had been operated on before the arthroplasty. With no elbow operations before arthroplasty, the risk of ulnar symptoms was 10%; with previous operations the risk was 24%. Bone resorption of a variable degree was noted in osteoporotic joints. Thirty-nine patients were satisfied with the result of the surgery; 13 were not. Sixteen considered the results "good," 32 "satisfactory," and 3 "bad." Forty-four patients said they would have the operation again.

These studies illustrate that cutis has proved to be a successful autogenous interposing membrane in arthroplasties. Cutis is strong, pliable, and well tolerated by the host, and has exhibited few negative results. However, the popularity of cutis seems to have declined since the advent of biologic allograft scaffolds.

Burkhead and colleagues[10,11] described the resurfacing of the glenohumeral joint with an acellular regenerative tissue scaffold. In 2008, Berlet and colleagues[12] detailed the interpositional arthroplasty of the first metatarsophalangeal (MTP) joint in 9 patients with a 12-month follow-up. Increased function and a reduction in pain were attributed to the scaffold's ability to maintain the inherent nature of the joint and the resurfacing of the first metatarsal-sesamoid articulation. Also in 2008, Lee described the resurfacing of the tibio-talar joint with the use of external fixation and an acellular regenerative tissue (ART) scaffold. At a minimum of 8 months, 18 ankles exhibited increased function and decreased pain.[13]

The purpose of this article is to describe additional cases in which the ankle and first MTP joint underwent biologic resurfacing, with a 2-year postoperative follow-up.

ACELLULAR HUMAN DERMAL SCAFFOLD

The ART scaffold (Graftjacket, Wright Medical Technology, Arlington, TN) is a type of acellular human dermal scaffold that can be used to treat tendon and ligament injuries, as well as full-thickness skin wounds. ART is an allogeneic permanent dermal equivalent derived from human cadaveric tissue, and is processed in a way that minimizes the destruction of the original human dermis.[14] This process preserves the extracellular matrix that contains elastin, proteoglycans, laminin, tenacin, and collagen types I, III, IV, and VIII; it also preserves the vascular channels of the cadaveric dermis (**Fig. 1**).[15] However, the main objective of the processing technique is to remove all immunogenic components and preserve the extracellular scaffold; this allows for rapid revascularization and cellular repopulation, and maintains tensile strength.

In the operative setting, the surgeon will notice that the scaffold contains 2 sides: the *active side* and the *basement membrane surface*. The active side—the side that will be applied to the augmented tissue—is called the *reticular surface*. The reticular surface is the intact collagen network that will serve as the scaffold for revascularization and cellular repopulation. The reticular surface incorporates into, and is gradually

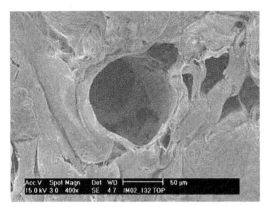

Fig.1. Electron scanning microscopy image of the acellular regenerative tissue (ART) scaffold and its intact vascular channel. (*Reprinted courtesy of* Wright Medical Technology, Arlington, TN; with permission.)

reorganized by, the host tissue. The other side of the scaffold, the basement membrane surface, is the anatomic equivalent of the epidermal-dermal junction, and will resorb as the reticular surface becomes populated by host cells (**Fig. 2**).

The load-failure strength of acellular human dermis scaffold was assessed by Barber and colleagues[16] in 2006. Compared with other commercially available allografts and xenografts,[16] the acellular human dermis (ie, ART) was found to have superior tensile load strength and suture retention. This benefit was attributed to the preservation of the human extracellular matrix during processing.[16,17]

The acellular human dermis scaffold minimizes host immune response while providing enough strength to withstand the shear forces of the foot and ankle joints.[10–13] These characteristics make the acellular human dermis scaffold an effective choice for biologic resurfacing.

DISTRACTION ARTHROPLASTY WITH TALAR RESURFACING

A 56-year-old man presents with an extremely painful arthritic ankle and a history of right distal tibia-fibula fracture 33 years before presentation (**Fig. 3**). Opposed to ankle fusion and unsure about total ankle arthroplasty due to "limited data," the patient consents to distraction arthroplasty with talar resurfacing.

An external fixator device is applied to the ankle and leg for distraction of the tibiotalar joint. The authors prefer a strong monolateral device to better access the anterior

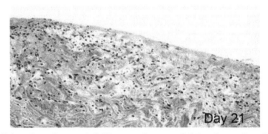

Fig. 2. Histologic slide of nude rat Achilles tendon model 21 days after implantation. Slide demonstrates tenocyte proliferation across the collagen scaffold.

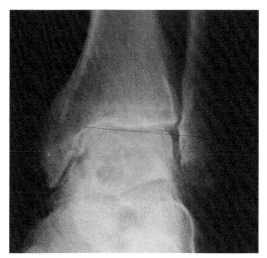

Fig. 3. Preoperative radiograph of severe tibio-talar joint arthritis before biologic resurfacing.

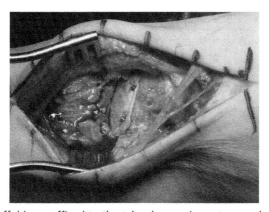

Fig. 4. Anterior ankle exposure after the joint distraction has occurred.

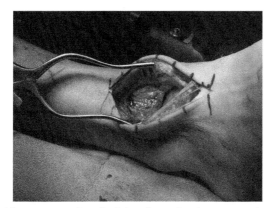

Fig. 5. The ART scaffold was affixed to the talar dome using suture anchors.

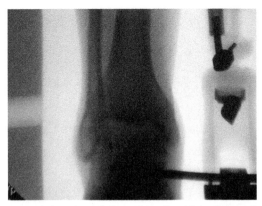

Fig. 6. Immediate postoperative view of the ankle after biologic resurfacing.

aspect of the ankle during the resurfacing approach. Using the fixator, the tibio-talar joint is distracted approximately 1 cm.

A standard anterior approach is used to access the tibio-talar joint. Attention initially is directed to the superficial peroneal nerve deep to the skin. Blunt dissection is carried to the deep tissue, where the neurovascular bundle is visualized and protected (**Fig. 4**). Once seen, attention is directed to the anterior lip of the tibia and extra-articular structures. A complete cheilectomy of the ankle is performed. While performing the joint debridement, the acellular human dermal bioscaffold is soaking in a warm bath of sterile saline. This material is properly hydrated when the paper attached to the scaffold is easily removed.

Once the extra-articular joint structures are debrided, the articular surface of the talar dome is prepared. The entire dorsal aspect of the talar dome is debrided to bleeding subchondral bone, and the acellular human dermal bioscaffold is cut to match the size of the dome. Using an anterior-to-posterior pattern of suture anchors, this material is affixed to the talar dome with the reticular surface facing toward the exposed subchondral bone (**Fig. 5**). It is important to ensure that the bioscaffold is affixed smoothly to the talar dome, as any folds or creases may disrupt the incorporation of the scaffold (**Fig. 6**).

Postoperatively the patient is encouraged to engage in as much weight bearing as possible. Van Roermund and colleagues[18] hypothesized that weight bearing during distraction allows for changes in intra-articular fluid pressure and an increase in synovial fluid production. This activity, coupled with a decrease in shear force across the joint, allows for reparative activity to occur in osteoarthritic cartilage.

Table 1 Pain scale				
Pain Scale (0–10)	**Preop.**	**6 months**	**1 year**	**2 years**
First step out of bed	9	4	3	0
Pain when standing	8	3	0	0
Pain when walking	9	4	2	0
Pain at the end of the day	9	5	3	1

Pain scale: 0 is no pain, 10 equals worst pain possible.

Table 2
Function scale

Function Scale (0–10)	Preop.	6 months	1 year	2 years
When climbing stairs	9	6	2	0
When descending stairs	9	5	3	1
When standing tiptoe	9	6	3	1
When running	10	10	10	10

Function scale: 0 is no difficulty, 10 equals unable to perform.

The fixator is removed at 3 months, and the patient is placed in a rigorous physical therapy program to address functional and mechanical instability, strength, and range of motion. The data given in **Tables 1–3** describe pain, function, and assistant device at 6 months, 1 year, and 2 years postoperatively.

FIRST METATARSAL HEAD BIOLOGIC RESURFACING WITH HEMI-ARTHROPLASTY

A 52-year-old woman with prior first MTP joint hemi-arthroplasty presents with joint pain, limited range of motion, and jamming. Radiographs demonstrate a hemi-implant in poor position with a significant decrease in first MTP joint space. This patient consents to biologic resurfacing of the first metatarsal, with a goal of decreasing pain, increasing range of motion, addressing the degeneration of the first metatarsal head, and using the acellular human dermal bioscaffold (Graftjacket, Wright Medical Technology, Arlington, TN) as a separating medium between the first metatarsal-sesamoid complex.

A linear incision is created over the course of the first MTP joint. To expose the first metatarsal head, dissection is carried to the level of the joint. The metatarsal head is debrided, removing all extra-articular spurs and releasing the sesamoid-first metatarsal complex. Using a cup-and-cone reaming system, the first metatarsal head is shaped using the conical reamer (**Fig. 7**). Reaming occurs to the level of subchondral, bleeding bone. All articular cartilage is removed. The base of the proximal phalanx is prepared for hemi-arthroplasty with a cup reamer and sagittal saw (**Fig. 8**). During the debridement of the first MTP joint, the bioscaffold is soaked in a warm bath of sterile saline.

Using a 2.0 drill bit, 2 vertical trephine holes are drilled into the metaphyseal region of the first metatarsal (**Fig. 9**). Using a strong, nonabsorbable suture, the human dermal bioscaffold is tagged, and then passed through each of the trephine holes with a tendon passer (**Fig. 10**). The bioscaffold is wrapped around the metatarsal head in a "hoodlike" fashion. The nonabsorbable suture is then sewn around the metatarsal neck using an "under-and-over" technique (**Fig. 11**). The excess

Table 3
Assistant device

Assistant Device	Preop.	6 months	1 year	2 years
Use indoors	7	4	0	0
Use outdoors	8	5	0	0

Assistant Device Scale: 0 is never use, 10 is use all of the time.

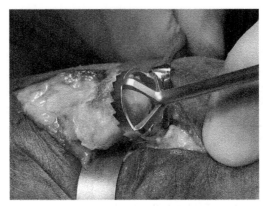

Fig. 7. Preparation of the first metatarsal head using conical reamer.

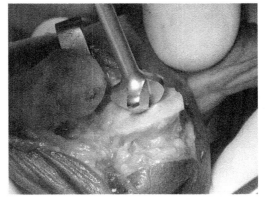

Fig. 8. Preparation of the base of the proximal phalanx for hemiarthroplasty.

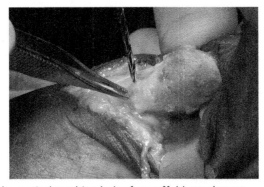

Fig. 9. Drilling of the vertical trephine holes for scaffold attachment.

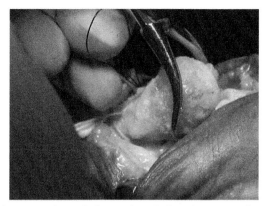

Fig. 10. Passing of the suture through the trephine holes. This action allows for proper placement of the scaffold on the metatarsal head.

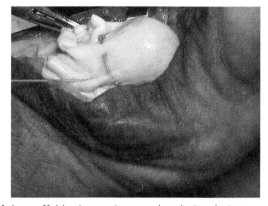

Fig. 11. Suturing of the scaffold using an "over and under" technique.

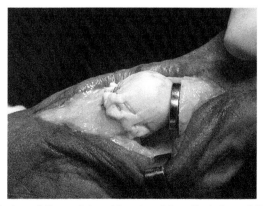

Fig. 12. Final resurfacing of the metatarsal head and its articulation of the hemi-implant.

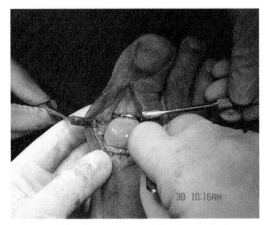

Fig. 13. Intraoperative view of the first metatarsal head resurfacing.

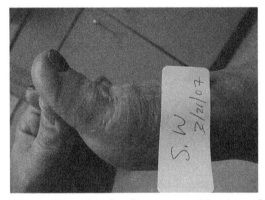

Fig. 14. Great to dorsiflexion 6 months after first metatarsal head resurfacing.

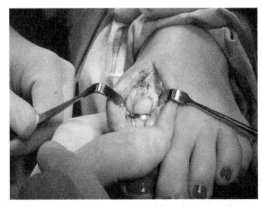

Fig. 15. Intraoperative views of the first metatarsal head previously resurfaced.

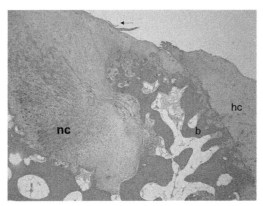

Fig. 16. Host cartilage (hc) is present above the subchondral bone (b). The cartilage surface is irregular and adjacent, and there is loss of articular cartilage (*arrow*). Neocartilage (nc) is present (hematoxylin-eosin, original magnification ×10).

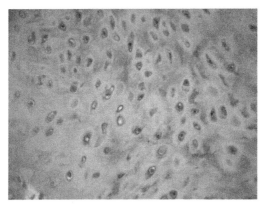

Fig. 17. Higher magnification of neocartilage reveals mature, differentiated chondrocytes with dense proteoglycan deposition (hematoxylin-eosin, original magnification ×40).

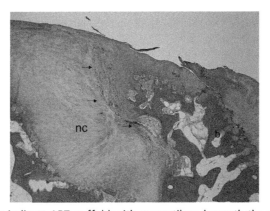

Fig. 18. The arrows indicate ART scaffold with neocartilage beneath the scaffold (nc). Subchondral bone (b) is adjacent to the newly formed cartilage.

bioscaffold is removed, and the hemi-implant is placed in the base of the proximal phalanx (**Figs. 12** and **13**).

During postoperative examination the patient was found to have less pain and more function (**Fig. 14**). Eighteen months postoperatively, the patient presented with tenderness to the first interspace, and biopsy of the previously resurfaced metatarsal head was performed. Visual inspection demonstrated an articular surface with smooth, shiny, "hyaline-like" appearance (**Fig. 15**). Histologic analysis showed a significant layer of neocartilage adjacent to the subchondral bone (**Fig. 16**). Higher magnification of the neocartilage revealed mature, differentiated chondrocytes throughout the matrix of the acellular human dermal bioscaffold (**Figs. 17** and **18**). These findings confirm that the bioscaffold is able to accept host chondrocytes and form a joint surface that will act and function in a way similar to that of articular cartilage.

SUMMARY

The goal of biologic resurfacing is to provide a smooth joint surface with a low coefficient of friction, which allows the joint to function with near-normal biomechanics, as well as provide intermittent pressure, to the subchondral and cancellous bone. This unique combination often results in the formation of a "neocartilage-like" structure that can reduce pain and restore biomechanics.

Due to its potential for regenerative healing, high tensile strength, and easy handling characteristics, acellular human dermal bioscaffold seems to be an excellent tissue for resurfacing. Although there has yet to be significant level 1 evidence that supports biologic resurfacing, the authors believe that as fixation techniques and technologies evolve, biologics will dominate the management of osteoarthritis.

REFERENCES

1. Baer WS. Arthroplasty with the aid of animal membrane. Am J Orthop Surg 1918; 16:1–29.
2. McKeever DC. The use of cellophane as an interposition membrane in synovectomy. J Bone Joint Surg Am 1943;25:576–80.
3. Burman MS. Plastic materials in medicine: preliminary report on the use of lucite and nylon fabric in orthopedic surgery. Am J Surg 1943;62:124–5.
4. Brown JE, McGaw WH, Shaw DT. Use of cutis as an interposing membrane in arthroplasty of the knee. J Bone Joint Surg Am 1958;40:1003–18.
5. Kettunen K. Changes in the fresh autogenous whole-thickness skin graft used as interposition material in arthroplasty of the hip joint on cats: preliminary report. Ann Chir Gynaecol Fenn 1956;45:193–6.
6. Kelley JW, Gross WM. Dermal arthroplasty of the hip joint. Plast Reconstr Surg 1959;23:540–6.
7. Bailey BN. Dermal arthroplasty. Hand 1971;3:135–7.
8. Froimson AI, Silva JE, Richey DG. Cutis arthroplasty of the elbow joint. J Bone Joint Surg Am 1976;58:863–5.
9. Uuspää V. Anatomical interposition arthroplasty with dermal graft. A study of 51 elbow arthroplasties on 48 rheumatoid patients. Z Rheumatol 1987;46:132–5 [in Finnish].
10. Burkhead WZ, Krishnan SG, Lin KC. Biologic resurfacing of the arthritic glenohumeral joint: historical review and current applications. J Shoulder Elbow Surg 2007;16(5):248–53.
11. Krishnan SG, Reineck JR, Burkhead WZ. Biological resurfacing of the glenoid in the athlete. Oper Tech Sports Med 2008;16:26–31.

12. Berlet GC, Hyer CF, Lee TH, et al. Interpositional arthroplasty of the first metatar-sophalangeal joint using a regenerative tissue matrix for the treatment of advanced hallux rigidus. Foot Ankle Int 2008;29(1):10–21.
13. Lee DK. Ankle arthroplasty alternatives with allograft and external fixation: prelim-inary clinical outcome. J Foot Ankle Surg 2008;47(5):447–52.
14. Callcut RA, Schurr MJ, Sloan M, et al. Clinical experience with Alloderm: a one-staged composite dermal/epidermal replacement utilizing processed cadaver dermis and thin autografts. Burns 2006;32:583–8.
15. Rubin L, Schweitzer S. The use of acellular biologic tissue patches in foot and ankle surgery. Clin Podiatr Med Surg 2005;22:533–52.
16. Barber FA, Herbert MA, Coons DA. Tendon augmentation grafts: biomechanical failure loads and failure patterns. Arthroscopy 2006;22(5):534–8.
17. Barber FA, McGarry JE, Herbert MA, et al. A biomechanical study of Achilles tendon repairs augmented with Graftjacket Matrix. Foot Ankle Int 2008;29(3): 329–33.
18. van Roermund PM, Marijnissen AC, Lafeber FP. Joint distraction as an alternative for the treatment of osteoarthritis. Foot Ankle Clin 2002;7(3):515–27.

Use of Soft Tissue Matrices as an Adjunct to Achilles Repair and Reconstruction

Brian S. Stover, DPM[a], Charles M. Zelen, DPM, FACFAS[b,c,d,*],
David L. Nielson, DPM[b]

KEYWORDS

• Xenograft • Achilles repair • Conexa • Orthobiologics

The Achilles tendon is the thickest and strongest tendon in the human body. In spite of this, it is also one of the most frequently ruptured tendons, accounting for nearly 40% of all surgically repaired tendons.[1] There have been many advancements in the repair of Achilles tendons since 1929 when Quénu and Stoïanovitch[2] advocated that rupture of the Achilles tendon should be operated on without delay. Over the last 15 years, there has been a drive to produce biologic and synthetic scaffolds to facilitate and strengthen the repair of ligamentous and tendinous injuries. Today many of these tendon grafts exist as autografts, allografts, xenografts, and synthetic materials. Even given these advancements, there remains much debate about the appropriate course of treatment for acute and chronic Achilles tendon ruptures.

Many early studies comparing surgical and conservative treatments favored a surgical treatment.[3,4] In the 1970s, Nisto[5] advocated a nonsurgical approach, stating that there was shorter morbidity time, fewer patient complaints, and no hospital stay. He found only minor differences between surgical and nonsurgical treatments. A cornerstone for the argument to choose conservative over surgical treatments was that surgery led to higher complication rates. Contrary to this, a review by Cetti and colleagues[6] showed that major complications occurred in 3.5% of the cases that were surgically repaired, compared with 18.1% in patients treated with

[a] Professional Education and Research Institute/SALSA, 222 Walnut Ave, Roanoke, VA 24016, USA
[b] Foot and Ankle Associates of Southwest Virginia, Professional Education and Research Institute, 222 Walnut Ave, Roanoke, VA 24016, USA
[c] Department of Surgery, Carilion Clinic, Roanoke, VA 24016, USA
[d] Department of Orthopedics, HCA Lewis Gale Hospital, Roanoke, VA 24016, USA
* Corresponding author. Professional Education and Research Institute, 222 Walnut Ave; Roanoke, VA 24016, USA.
E-mail address: cmzelen@periedu.com (C.M. Zelen).

Clin Podiatr Med Surg 26 (2009) 647–658
doi:10.1016/j.cpm.2009.08.011
0891-8422/09/$ – see front matter © 2009 Elsevier Inc. All rights reserved.

podiatric.theclinics.com

conservative therapies. Furthermore, the incidence of rerupture was higher in nonsurgically treated patients (13.4%) compared with surgically treated patients (1.4%).

Over the years, many operative methods have been proposed for the treatment of neglected Achilles tendon ruptures.[7] The types of repairs include, but are not limited to, augmented and nonaugmented repairs, percutaneous or minimally invasive repairs, and reconstructive repairs. Simple end-to-end and suture techniques are often inadequate for neglected repairs because of the deficit between ends that needs to be overcome. The ruptured Achilles can become so contracted as early as 3 to 4 days after rupture that end-to-end repair is not feasible.[8] In these instances, more advanced procedures involving soft tissue augmentation must be used. Many autogenously augmented procedures have been described including tendon transfers of the plantaris,[9] the flexor digitorum longus,[10] the flexor hallucis longus,[11] the peroneus brevis,[12] and gastrocnemius flaps in many varieties.[13–15]

The issues with these types of procedures are that they increase surgery and tourniquet time, are technically more difficult, decrease function and strength, require larger or multiple incisions, and may entail donor site morbidity.[16,17] It is for these reasons surgeons have turned to exogenous materials. Early trials with silk, Teflon, Silastic, and Silastic with Dacron were successful in proving that exogenous materials can be used to supplement tendon repairs.[13,18–20] In 1977, Jenkins and colleagues[21] used absorbable carbon fiber to repair tendons in sheep to induce new tendon growth. Synthetic materials were quite popular in the 1980s and early 1990s because of their mechanical characteristics. However, many of the materials had complications due to foreign body reactions, chronic inflammation, and osteolysis.[22]

It is for this reason a transition occurred to produce biologic grafts that are safe, stimulate very little host response, and integrate and degrade into the host tissues (ie, regenerate host tissues). The ideal graft material is sterile, nonreactive and converts or regenerates into the native tissue within 1 to 2 years.

Safety concerns regarding biologic grafts are centered on disease transmission and sterility. Human-derived allografts are required by the US Food and Drug Administration to screen and test donors for diseases such as HIV and hepatitis. Grafts are produced aseptically or sterilely. Aseptic processing and handling of the material is essential so that there is no introduction of additional bacteria. This does not necessarily mean that all bacteria is eradicated from the material. In order for a biologic medical device to be approved for implantation it must have a sterility assurance level (SAL) of 10^{-3}(1 in 1000 chance that material contains microbe). To be labeled as sterile, an SAL of 10^{-6} (1 in a million chance that material contains microbe) must be obtained.[23]

There are many reasons a biologic implant can produce a host response. Most notably are the presence of DNA material in the graft and the presence of a xenogeneic antigen (α-Gal). Remnant xenogeneic DNA has been implicated as the cause of severe inflammatory reactions.[24] Some xenogeneic scaffolds, including those derived from porcine small intestine submucosa (SIS), have been found to have high levels of α-Gal antigens. This antigen is found in most animal species with the exception of higher order species (humans and primates). In fact, humans produce large amounts of anti-Gal antibodies, which is a practical reason for many of these xenogeneic grafts to be rejected or mount an inflammatory response.[25]

Cross-linking of collagen implants may have a direct effect on their ability to facilitate tendon healing. Grafts that are cross-linked, chemically or naturally are resistant to enzymatic degradation and, therefore, more difficult to incorporate into the host tissues. As a result, the healing process is one of repair rather than regeneration. Reparative processes can create a weaker construct prone to failure because the body recognizes the graft as foreign and either breaks it down rapidly and fills it in with scar tissue, or encapsulates it. Encapsulation occurs because immune cells penetrate the graft's extracellular matrix making the graft unable to remodel. This often results in chronic inflammation consistent with a foreign body response.[26] Furthermore, cross-linking of materials may make the detection of DNA remnants and α-Gal antigens difficult.[25]

Conversely, materials with minimal cross-linking are subject to enzymatic degradation by the host. Cutting cones that penetrate the graft are followed by vascular budding, which ultimately leads to incorporation of the graft material by the host tissues. Instead of simply repairing the host tissue, properly degraded soft tissue matrices can be incorporated and contribute necessary components to help the tissues regenerate. Therefore, a graft that is capable of regeneration as opposed to reparation is preferred. Regeneration may occur with non–cross-linked grafts that are intact (nondamaged). The body accepts the graft and integrates the graft via revascularization and cell repopulation. Tissue that is regenerated is generally stronger compared with repaired or scarred tissue, and may be more similar to host tissues. Two commercially available soft tissue matrices, Graft Jacket (Wright Medical Technologies, Memphis, TN, USA) and Conexa (Tornier, Edina, MN, USA), are examples of three-dimensional scaffolds that are almost free of cross-linking caused by material preparation, and may allow for a regenerative repair via rapid revascularization and cellular population without the formation of scar tissue and encapsulation associated with its more heavily cross-linked counterparts.

The following case demonstrates how a soft tissue matrix can be used as a supplement to a complex Achilles repair. In this case, the authors will demonstrate the application of a soft tissue matrix to augment the repair.

CASE STUDY

A 70-year-old female presented with pain and weakness of the left, lower extremity after sustaining a fall. She had a history of diabetes and osteoporosis. Clinically there was absence of plantarflexion and a positive Thompson's test. On a radiograph, a clear avulsion of the Achilles was identified at the insertion (**Fig. 1**A), with remnant

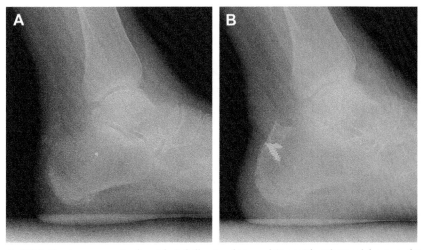

Fig. 1. (*A*) Patient preoperatively with Achilles tendon avulsion with calcaneal fracture fragments. (*B*) Patient 4-months status after successful surgical repair with soft tissue matrix.

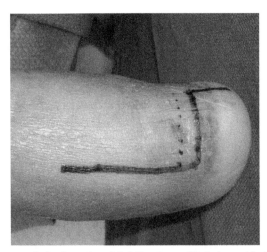

Fig. 2. Incisional approach for insertional Achilles tear with S-shaped incision.

bone fragments present on the ruptured tendon. Achilles repair and reattachment was recommended. An S-shaped incision was used (**Fig. 2**). The distal section of the tendon was freed of all nonviable calcaneal fracture fragments that were not repairable to the boney surface (**Fig. 3**). A modified Krakow suture technique was used to secure the tendon (**Fig. 4**). Significant retraction prevented reattachment in a neutral position; therefore, a gastrocnemius recession was performed to restore length (**Fig. 5**).

For this repair, we chose a collagen soft tissue matrix derived from porcine tissue. This material is essentially non–cross-linked. The soft tissue matrix (Conexa 200, Tornier, Edina, MN, USA) was soaked in a saline bath for a minimum of 2 minutes, and used to reinforce the gastrocnemius recession with number-two coated polyester suture using a modified lateral trap suture technique (**Fig. 5**). The Achilles was then

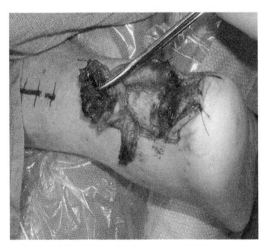

Fig. 3. Rupture of the distal Achilles from the insertion with fracture fragments of the calcaneus well visualized.

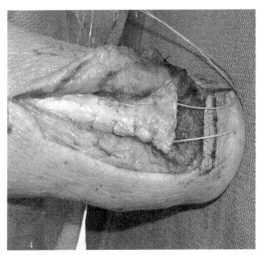

Fig. 4. Surgical repair with modified Krakow suture pattern. Significant retraction of the tendon was appreciated requiring adjunctive surgery to prevent significant talipes equinus.

anchored with titanium soft tissue anchors backed to the calcaneus (**Figs. 6** and **1B**), and the repair reinforced with a single posterior overlay of soft tissue matrix sutured with number-two coated polyester with a modified lateral trap suture technique (**Figs. 7** and **8**).

The patient was kept non-weight bearing for a period of 6 weeks, immobilized in a neutral 90 degree position. She then began gradual progress to activity. Full function

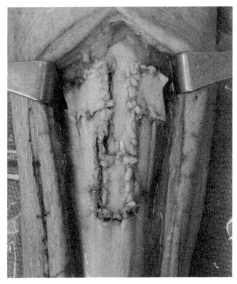

Fig. 5. Gastrocnemius resection with modified Baker tongue-and-groove demonstrated with the soft tissue matrix used to reinforce the tendon and cover the exposed muscle belly.

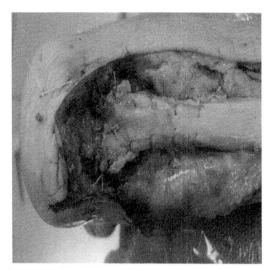

Fig. 6. Achilles tendon successfully anchored to posterior calcaneus.

was achieved of the Achilles tendon with minimal deficit and no soft tissue reaction was observed (**Fig. 9**).

DISCUSSION

Multiple soft tissue repair matrices are available with each one having distinctive biomechanical and resorptive capabilities. A group of xenografts exists that is derived from porcine SIS, including Restore and Cuffpatch. In 1999, Restore (DePuy Orthopedics, Warsaw, IN, USA) became the first biologic scaffold available commercially. Restore is a non–cross-linked, sterile patch that had early successes reported for

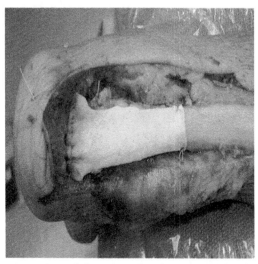

Fig. 7. Soft tissue matrix used to reinforce insertional repair. Initial tack stitches placed with 2-0–coated polyester suture.

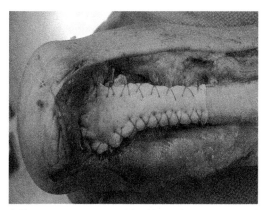

Fig. 8. Completed Achilles repair using a modified lateral trap suture technique to secure the soft tissue matrix into position.

its use in rotator cuff repairs.[27] However, later studies demonstrated that Restore was not suited for soft tissue repairs. Walton and colleagues[28] reported that 60% of patients treated for rotator cuff repairs with Restore patch had rerupture of their cuff, 6 to 24 months postoperatively. Subsequent studies reported severe postoperative edema following use of Restore patch.[29,30] It has been hypothesized that the problems associated with Restore may be the result of remnants of porcine DNA[25] and the α-Gal antigen[31] found in this material.

Cuffpatch (Organogenesis, Canton, MA, USA) is chemically cross-linked and is sterilized via gamma radiation. As discussed earlier, this added cross-linking may diminish the incorporation of the material into the host tissue because of increased resistance to enzymatic degradation. Cuffpatch was found to contain "negligible amounts of DNA."[32] However, it is porcine SIS which is contains α-Gal antigens. As expected, Cuffpatch was found to elicit a severe cellular response.[33] Additionally, when tested head-to-head with other patches, Cuffpatch was the weakest of those tested.[34] Cuffpatch is prehydrated, only requiring a rinse before use.

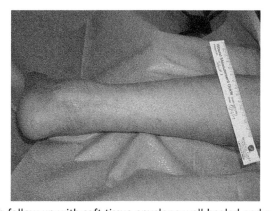

Fig. 9. Nine-month follow-up with soft tissue envelope well healed and no palpable prominence of soft tissue patch. No foreign body or soft reaction appreciated.

TissueMend (Stryker, Kalamazoo, MI, USA), and the ZCR (Zimmer, Warsaw, IN, USA) or Permacol (Covidien, Mansfield, MA, USA) patches, are derived from xenogeneic dermis. TissueMend is derived from fetal bovine dermis. The patch is aseptically processed and then sterilized in ethylene oxide. Seldes and Abramchayev[35] have reported that TissueMend has good strength, handling characteristics, storing capacity, and biocompatibility. TissueMend requires hydration of less than 1 minute. The ZCR patch is derived from porcine dermis. It is sterilized via gamma radiation. The ZCR patch has been successfully used in the reconstruction of abdominal walls, vaginal and urinary tracts, and, to some degree, in rotator cuff repairs.[23] The ZCR patch when tested against other grafts demonstrated good suture retention by resisting suture pull-through on the ends of the graft.[36] However, in several instances the patch is reported to have produced a noninfectious edema at the operative site.[36,37] This may be because this patch has one of the slowest degradation rates compared with other patches and may become completely encapsulated by the human body.[35] It may also be associated with α-Gal antigens. The ZCR patch requires no hydration.

OrthAdapt (Pegasus Biologics, Irvine, CA, USA) is a cross-linked scaffold derived from equine pericardium. There are only a few case studies available regarding OrthAdapt.[38–41] In a study funded by Pegasus Biologics, OrthAdapt was compared with Cuffpatch and found to be biomechanically equivalent.[42] However, Cuffpatch is a poor comparator as it has been shown to be the weakest of five tested scaffolds.[36] Most recently, significant foreign body reactions have been reported anecdotally with the use of OrthAdapt; the overall incidence of these reactions and the cause are unknown.

Graftjacket (Wright Medical Technology, Arlington, TN, USA) was introduced for orthopedic procedures in 2002. Graftjacket is a non–cross-linked allograft derived from human cadaver skin. It is aseptically processed and has been shown to be regenerative in nature. Graftjacket has been used successfully in the treatment of ulcers and orthopedic procedures. The first case reports of using Graftjacket for Achilles repairs appeared in 2004,[43] with multiple studies following. Biomechanically, Graftjacket was found to be superior in terms of failure force compared with four other products (Permacol or ZCR, Cuffpatch, TissueMend, and Restore).[36] Another study, done in 2008 by Barber and colleagues,[44] took eight matched pairs of cadaver legs and simulated Achilles ruptures. All legs were repaired via a Krakow stitch and one of each pair was augmented with Graftjacket. It was reported that the legs augmented with Graftjacket had, on average, twice the failure load compared with the control (control ultimate failure load was 217 N $\pm$ 31 compared with 455 N $\pm$ 76.5 with Graftjacket). Graftjacket is human-derived and, therefore, an antigenic response to α-Gal is nonexistent. However, Graftjacket still maintains a relatively high level of DNA content. In fact, Graftjacket is the only scaffold that contains full DNA strands, whereas all others contain remnants.[45] This may explain why Graftjacket elicited a more intense acute cellular response when compared with other biologic scaffolds.[45] As mentioned, Graftjacket is only aseptically processed, not sterile. Although this may raise concerns of disease transmission, there have been no cases reported which demonstrate that diseases have been transmitted by this product. Graftjacket requires a minimum 5-minute hydration and requires specific orientation requirements for proper application.

Conexa (Conexa Reconstructive Tissue Matrix, Tornier, Edina, MN, USA) is a sterile xenograft derived from porcine dermis. Conexa is non–cross-linked and, therefore, supports a regenerative process of host tissues encouraging healing and prevents the formation of scar tissue and encapsulation that can inhibit native cellular

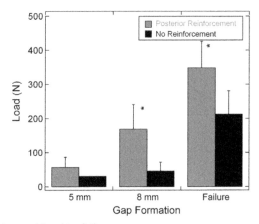

Fig. 10. Gap formation and load-to-failure.

repopulation and vascular in-growth. The processing of Conexa significantly reduces the α-Gal antigen responsible for xenogeneic response. In addition to supporting incorporation without inflammatory reaction, Conexa has been found in biomechanical studies to show superior strength. Six matched pairs of fresh frozen legs underwent complete transection of the Achilles tendon. One specimen from each matched pair was repaired with a Krakow stitch and the contralateral side was repaired with a Krakow stitch followed by augmentation with Conexa. All specimens were then cyclically loaded to test for gap formation. It was reported that four out of the six Krakow-only specimens had a greater than 8 mm gap formation under cyclic loading (<30N), whereas none of the Conexa-reinforced group specimens had 8 mm gap formation under cyclic loading. Furthermore, the Conexa-reinforced group had significantly higher load-to-failure as compared with the non-reinforced group ($348 \pm 78N$ vs $212 \pm 68N$) (**Figs. 10** and **11**).

Suture retention strength was also compared with many of the commercially available grafts and both Conexa and Graftjacket were found to have superior suture

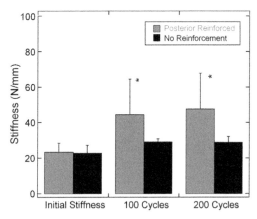

Fig. 11. Repair stiffness.

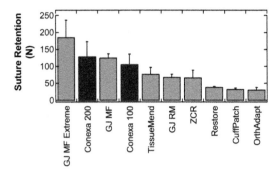

Fig. 12. Suture retention strength of various soft tissue matrices. (*From* Walton JR, Bowman NK, Khatib Y, Linklater J, Murrell, GA. Restore orthobiologic implant: not recommended for augmentation of rotator cuff repairs. J Bone Joint Surg Am 2007;89(4):786–91; with permission.)

retention strength when compared with the other available soft tissue repair matrices (**Fig. 12**). Because of the superior strength, excellent incorporation into host tissues, and minimal complications associated with host responses, this material performed optimally for the repair. Furthermore, it is available in two thicknesses, allowing the surgeon to tailor its use for a variety of applications.

SUMMARY

In this article, the Conexa soft tissue matrix is shown to be a viable solution for Achilles tendon repairs with early studies showing superior biomechanical strength and biocompatibility. The authors' experience with this product further validates this early data with a case study of an Achilles repair showing soft tissue matrices as a successful adjunct to both the primary repair and gastrocnemius recession, with full return to activity and no inflammatory response appreciated at long-term follow up. The authors anticipate that the use of soft tissue matrices for the repair of tendon and soft tissue defects will expand over time. This material has distinct advantages over synthetics and highly cross-linked biologic materials, which can trigger host responses and associated complications.

REFERENCES

1. Jozsa L, Kvist M, Balint BJ, et al. The role of recreational sport activity in Achilles tendon rupture: a clinical, pathoanatomical, and sociological study of 292 cases. Am J Sports Med 1989;17:338–43.
2. Quénu J, Stoïanovitch. Les ruptures du tendon d'Achilles [Rupture of Achilles tendon]. Rev Chir Paris 1929;67:647–78 [in French].
3. Arner O, Lindholm Å. Subcutaneous rupture of the Achilles tendon. Acta Chir Scand 1959;239:7–51.
4. Christensen IB. Rupture of the Achilles tendon: analysis of 57 cases. Acta Chir Scand 1953;106:50–60.
5. Nistor L. Surgical and non-surgical treatment of Achilles tendon rupture. J Bone Joint Surg Am 1981;63:394–9.
6. Cetti R, Christensen SE, Ejsted R, et al. Operative versus nonoperative treatment of Achilles tendon rupture. Am J Sports Med 1993;21:791–9.

7. Gabel S, Manoli A. Neglected Achilles tendon rupture. Foot Ankle 1994;15:512–7.
8. Bosworth DM. Repair of defects in the tendo Achillis. J Bone Joint Surg Am 1956; 38:111–4.
9. Lynn TA. Repair of the torn Achilles tendon, using the Plantaris tendon as a reinforcing membrane. J Bone Joint Surg Am 1966;48:268–72.
10. Mann RA, Holmes GP, Seale KS, et al. Chronic rupture of the Achilles tendon: a new technique of repair. J Bone Joint Surg Am 1991;73:214–9.
11. Wapner KL, Hecht PJ, Mills RH Jr. Reconstruction of neglected Achilles tendon injury. Orthop Clin North Am 1995;26:249–63.
12. Teuffeur AP. Traumatic rupture of the Achilles tendon: reconstruction by transplant and graft using the lateral peroneus brevis. Orthop Clin North Am 1974;5:89–93.
13. Williams RD. Teflon as a tendon substitute. Surg Forum 1960;11:39–40.
14. Mahmoud SW, Megahed AA, Sheshtawy OE. Repair of the calcaneal tendon: an improved technique. J Bone Joint Surg Am 1992;74:114–7.
15. Chen DS, Wertheimer SJ. A new method of repair for rupture of the Achilles tendon. J Foot Surg 1992;31:440–5.
16. Pajala A, Kangas J, Siira P, et al. Augmented compared with nonaugmented surgical repair of a fresh total Achilles tendon rupture. A Prospective Randomized Study. J Bone Joint Surg Am 2009;91:1092–100.
17. Lee DK. Achilles tendon repair with acellular tissue graft augmentation in neglected ruptures. J Foot Ankle Surg 2007;46(6):451–5.
18. Henze CW, Mayer L. An experimental study of silk-tendon plastics with particular reference to the prevention of post-operative adhesions. Surg Gynecol Obstet 1914;19:10–24.
19. Bader KF, Curtin JW. A successful silicone tendon prosthesis. Arch Surg 1968;97: 406–11.
20. Salisbury RF, Mason AD Jr, Levin NS, et al. Artificial tendons: design, application and results. J Trauma 1974;14:580–6.
21. Jenkins DHR, Foster IW, McKibbin B, et al. Induction of tendon and ligament formation by carbon implants. J Bone Joint Surg Br 1977;59:53–7.
22. Chen J, Xu J, Wang A, et al. Scaffolds for tendon and ligament repair: review of the efficacy of commercial products. Expert Rev Med Devices 2009;6(1):61–73.
23. Updated 510(k) Sterility Review Guidance K90-1: Final Guidance for Industry and FDA. Food and Drug Administration; 2002. Available at: www.fda.gov. Accessed September 2, 2009.
24. Zheng MH, Chen J, Kirilak Y, et al. Porcine small intestine submucosa (SIS) is not an acellular collagenous matrix and contains porcine DNA: possible implications in human implantation. J Biomed Mater Res B Appl Biomater 2005;73:61–7.
25. Badylak SF, Gilbert TW. Immune response to biologic scaffold materials. Semin Immunol 2008;20(2):109–16.
26. Sandor M, Xu H, Connor J, et al. Host response to implanted porcine-derived biologic materials in a primate model of abdominal wall repair. Tissue Eng Part A 2008;14(12):2021–31.
27. Metcalf MH, Savoie F, Kelluma B. Surgical technique for xenograft (SIS) augmentation of rotator-cuff repairs. Oper Tech Orthopaedics 2002;12(3):204–8.
28. Walton JR, Bowman NK, Khatib Y, et al. Restore orthobiologic implant: not recommended for augmentation of rotator cuff repairs. J. Bone Joint Surg Am 2007; 89(4):786–91.
29. Malcarney HL, Bonar F, Murrell GA. Early inflammatory reaction after rotator cuff repair with porcine small intestine submucosal implants: a report of 4 cases. Am J Sports Med 2005;33(6):907–11.

30. Iannotti JP, Codsi MJ, Kwan YW, et al. Porcine small intestine submucosa augmentation of surgical repair of chronic two-tendon rotator cuff tears. A randomized, controlled trial. J Bone Joint Surg Am 2006;88(6):1238–44.

31. McPherson TB, Liang H, Record RD, et al. Galalpha(1,3)Gal epitope in porcine small intestinal submucosa. Tissue Eng 2000;6:233–9.

32. Derwin KA, Baker AR, Spragg RK, et al. Commercial extracellular matrix scaffolds for rotator cuff tendon repair. Biomechanical, biochemical, and cellular properties. J Bone Joint Surg Am 2006;88:2665–72.

33. Valentin JE, Badylak JS, McCabe GP, et al. Extracellular matrix bioscaffolds for orthopaedic applications. A comparative histologic study. J Bone Joint Surg Am 2006;88(12):2673–86.

34. Barber FA, Herbert MA, Coons DA. Tendon augmentation grafts: biomechanical failure loads and failure patterns. Arthroscopy 2006;22:534–8.

35. Seldes RM, Abramchayev I. Arthroscopic insertion of a biologic rotator cuff tissue augmentation after rotator cuff repair. Arthroscopy 2006;22(1):113–6.

36. Soler JA, Gidwani S, Curtis MJ. Early complications from the use of porcine dermal collagen implants (Permacol) as bridging constructs in the repair of 4 cases. Acta Orthop Belg 2007;73(4):432–6.

37. Belcerh JH, Zic R. Adverse effect of porcine collagen interposition after trapeziecetomy: a comparative study. J Hand Surg 2001;26(2):159–64.

38. Weil L Jr, Kuruvilla B, Bergman D, et al. Pegasus OrthAdapt Bioimplant: A Novel Approach to Hallux Varus Correction. Available at: www.Weil4Feet.com. Accessed July 17, 2009.

39. Fridman R, Cain JD, Weil L Jr. Augmented Bröstrom Repair Using Biologic Collagen Implant: Report on 9 Consecutive Patients. Foot Ankle 2008;1(7):4.

40. Lewicky Y, Tasto JP. Case Study: OrthAdapt Bioimplant used for Acromoclavicular joint recontruction. 2007.

41. Lefkowitz H. Case Study: OrthAdapt Bioimplant provides excellent scaffold for posterior tibial tendon repair. 2007.

42. Johnson W, Inamasu J, Yantzer B, et al. Comparative in vitro biomechanical evaluation of two soft tissue defect products. J. Biomed. Mater. Res. B. Appl. Biomater 2007.

43. Lee MS. Graftjacket augmentation of chronic Achilles tendon ruptures. Available at: www.orthosupersite.com/print.asp?rID=2305. Accessed July 13, 2009.

44. Barber FA, McGarry JE, Herbert MA, et al. A biomechanical study of Achilles tendon repair augmentation using GraftJacket matrix. Foot Ankle Int 2008; 23(3):329–33.

45. Xu H, Wan H, Sandor M, et al. Host response to human acellular dermal matrix transplantation in a primate model of abdominal wall repair. Tissue Eng Part A 2008;14(12):2009–19.

Index

Note: Page numbers of article titles are in **boldface** type.

A

Acellular dermal allografts
    for arthroplasty, 633–642
    for plantar soft tissue augmentation, **543–555**
Achilles tendon repair
    extracellular matrix biomaterials for, 516–517
    soft tissue matrices for, **645–656**
Adaptation, to extracellular matrix biomaterials, 514–515
Adoption, of extracellular matrix biomaterials, 514–515
Alloderm biomaterial, 512
Allografts, bone, 590–594, 598
AlloMax biomaterial, 507
AlloPatch biomaterial, 507
Apligraf living skin equivalent, 528–530
ART scaffold, for arthroplasty, 633–642
Arthrodesis, bone growth stimulation for, 611–613
Arthroplasty, **631–643**
    acellular human dermal scaffold for, 633–634
    distraction, with talar resurfacing, 634–637
    hemi-, with first metatarsal head resurfacing, 637–642
    history of, 631–633

B

Bioblanket, for tendon repair, 536
Bioscaffolds
    collagen, 525–527
    for arthroplasty, 633–642
    for ligament repair, 535–539
    for tendon repair, 535–539
Biostep collagen products, 524
Bone grafts and bone graft substitutes, **587–603**
    allografts, 590–594, 598
    cell-based, 596, 599
    classification of, 587–588
    factor-based, 596, 599
    processing of, 588–590
    synthetic, 595–598
    xenografts, 594–595, 598
Bone growth stimulation, **605–616**
    biology of, 606

Clin Podiatr Med Surg 26 (2009) 659–665
doi:10.1016/S0891-8422(09)00094-9
0891-8422/09/$ – see front matter © 2009 Elsevier Inc. All rights reserved.

podiatric.theclinics.com

Moving?

Make sure your subscription moves with you!

To notify us of your new address, find your **Clinics Account Number** (located on your mailing label above your name), and contact customer service at:

Email: journalscustomerservice-usa@elsevier.com

800-654-2452 (subscribers in the U.S. & Canada)
314-447-8871 (subscribers outside of the U.S. & Canada)

Fax number: 314-447-8029

Elsevier Health Sciences Division
Subscription Customer Service
3251 Riverport Lane
Maryland Heights, MO 63043

*To ensure uninterrupted delivery of your subscription, please notify us at least 4 weeks in advance of move.

Printed and bound by CPI Group (UK) Ltd, Croydon, CR0 4YY

03/10/2024

01040450-0018